Gluten-Free Cooking

More Than 150 Gluten-Free Recipes

Ruby M. Brown

T0273568

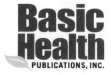

Basic Health
PUBLICATIONS, INC.

The information contained in this book is based upon the research and personal and professional experiences of the author. It is not intended as a substitute for consulting with your physician or other healthcare provider. Any attempt to diagnose and treat an illness should be done under the direction of a healthcare professional.

The publisher does not advocate the use of any particular healthcare protocol but believes the information in this book should be available to the public. The publisher and author are not responsible for any adverse effects or consequences resulting from the use of the suggestions, preparations, or procedures discussed in this book. Should the reader have any questions concerning the appropriateness of any procedures or preparation mentioned, the author and the publisher strongly suggest consulting a professional healthcare advisor.

Basic Health Publications, Inc.
28812 Top of the World Drive
Laguna Beach, CA 92651
949-715-7327 • www.basichealthpub.com

Published by arrangement with Sally Milner Publishing,
Bowral, New South Wales, Australia.

Library of Congress Cataloging-in-Publication Data

Brown, Ruby M.
    Gluten-free cooking : more than 150 gluten-free recipes / Ruby M. Brown.
      p. cm.
    Includes bibliographical references and index.
    ISBN 978-1-59120-202-8
  1. Gluten-free diet—Recipes. 2. Celiac disease—Diet therapy—Recipes.
3. Wheat-free diet—Recipes. I. Title.

    RM237.86.B7663   2007
    641.5'638—dc22

                        2007005646

Editor: Tara Durkin
Typesetting/Book design: Gary A. Rosenberg
Cover design: Mike Stromberg

Printed in the United States of America

10 9 8 7 6 5 4 3 2 1

Contents

Acknowledgments, iv

Foreword, v

Preface, vi

PART I • PRINCIPLES OF A GLUTEN-FREE DIET

1. Eating Well on a Gluten-Free Diet—
A Dietitian's Perspective, 3

2. Dietary Principles, 9

3. Celiac Disease and Gluten-Free Diets, 13

PART II • RECIPES

Measurements and Conversion Tables, 26

4. Breakfast, 29

5. Soups and Starters, 39

6. Main Courses, 55

7. Salads and Vegetables, 93

8. Desserts, 121

9. Holiday Fare, 143

10. Goodies to Bake, 157

11. Bread, Sweet Loaves, Muffins, and Extras, 187

Glossary, 237

Index, 246

About the Author, 250

Acknowledgments

I WISH TO EXPRESS MY MOST SINCERE THANKS and appreciation to my family and others who have made many contributions to the publication of this book:

To my precious husband, Kevin, for all the time, love, and understanding you have expressed in our home while this book was being written. Without your untiring support for my work as an author, this book would not have been possible.

To my daughters, Angela-Mary Bowden and Maria Manton, to whom I am devoted. Thank you for your contributions to this book. Your continued interest in the preparation of special diets has been evidenced by the number of recipes you have helped me to compile. Maria has also contributed in her capacity as a dietitian, with professional information on the daily management of a gluten-free diet.

To Penny, Lois, and Denise who were ever willing to be my taste-testers each week as new recipes were developed.

To Cheryl Price (Coeliac Society of Australia, Inc.) for her expertise in relation to celiac disease and for her interest in my work.

To Judy Wellins, consultant dietitian, for the foreword and her critiquing of my work.

To Roma Food Products for their products for developing recipes.

To Cooking Co-ordinates at Belconnen Fresh Food Markets in Canberra, Australia, where I regularly make guest appearances demonstrating and lecturing in special diets, particularly gluten-free diets.

Foreword

HERE ARE OUR FAVORITE, "TRADITIONAL" RECIPES, modified where required to suit the individual with celiac disease (or needing to avoid gluten protein) and reflecting the current interest in eating for overall health.

These recipes are gluten-free and have been reduced in fat, salt, and sugar where necessary, and boosted with fiber where possible. Butter is used in some recipes because a particular flavor is preferred. However the option is given to use mono- or polyunsaturated margarine/fats. The choice is yours.

Most important, the flavor and result of Ruby's gluten-free products have kept the quality of the original-style recipe, as best as possible (maybe even better!).

This book is another showcase of Ruby's natural flair for cooking and her interest in maintaining good health. She teaches healthy eating principles, including "special diets" and recipe modification, as part of health and weight-control programs. Ruby always impresses the participants with unique and interesting ways to "play" with recipes—for a healthier result.

Ruby is a multitalented culinary author and food technology educator. Her niche, as an author, is in the area of special diets, where she has published a variety of books, including *Good Food for Diabetes, Healthy Country Cooking, Wheat-Free Cooking,* and *Milk-Free Cooking.* Adding to Ruby's impressive range of successful writing are student textbooks and a craft book, *Decorated Eggs.*

Here is Ruby Brown's new collection of recipes, all free from gluten and delicious. Share the experience with your family and friends.

Judy Wellins B.Sc. (Nutr.), M.Sc. (Nutr. & Diet.),
Accredited Practicing Dietitian (Australia)

Preface

I HAVE WRITTEN *GLUTEN-FREE COOKING* through my personal experience, to help people who have been diagnosed with celiac disease. The sudden need to introduce a special diet into your family can often at first be very daunting. I hope *Gluten-Free Cooking* will help you to carefully undertake the planning of meals with as little concern as possible, and to enjoy gluten-free food. I trust you will be encouraged as you face the special dietary requirements that at first may seem like a crisis in your life. Remember, there is life after being diagnosed with celiac disease. Many of my readers are living proof of this.

This book is designed to help you with your special dietary requirements. As a celiac, your digestive system is damaged by gluten. This, then, makes it necessary for you to make a lifetime commitment to follow a gluten-free diet, with no exceptions to the rule.

Recipes for those on a gluten-free diet have in the past been a little dull. Today, with such a wide variety of gluten-free products readily available, it is possible to plan interesting meals using the recipes in this book.

The medical profession is now showing a greater awareness of celiac disease. Reliable medical tests have been developed to diagnose the condition. New ideas and developments in the area of gluten-free foods are occurring at a very rapid rate. Changes are happening even as this book is being written.

I recommend you join a celiac society or support group in your area. Celiac societies often provide ingredient lists, which are essential for those requiring a gluten-free diet, along with a lot of other helpful information. (To find your local celiac society or support group, please use the resources listed in Chapter 3.)

Ruby M. Brown

PART I
Principles of a Gluten-Free Diet

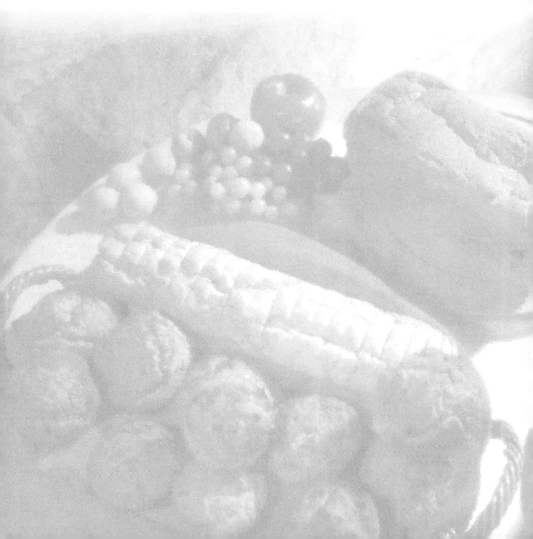

1.

Eating Well on a Gluten-Free Diet— A Dietitian's Perspective

by Maria Manton, B.Sc. (Nut.), M.Sc. (Nut. & Diet.),
Grad. Cert. Diab. Ed., Accredited Practicing Dietitian (Australia)

FOLLOWING A GLUTEN-FREE DIET IS ESSENTIAL in the management of celiac disease. A dietitian is professionally qualified to provide guidance and nutritional advice to ensure that a gluten-free eating plan is manageable as well as being nutritionally balanced.

THE LIFELONG DIET

When most people think of a "diet" they think of a short-term change in their eating pattern, but for those with celiac disease, a gluten-free diet should be continued throughout life. Having even small amounts of gluten in the diet may cause damage to the intestine. These small amounts may not produce symptoms immediately; however, damage to the intestine caused by any amount of gluten may lead to poor absorption of nutrients. This may result in deficiencies of nutrients such as calcium and iron. In the long term, continuing on a diet containing gluten substantially increases the risk of bowel cancer in someone with celiac disease.

HOW LONG IS IT NECESSARY TO REMAIN ON A GLUTEN-FREE DIET?

After gluten is removed from the diet, symptoms subside. The time for this varies between individuals. Someone with celiac disease will always be sensitive to gluten and as such they must remain on a gluten-free diet for life.

HEALTHY FOOD CHOICES ON
A GLUTEN-FREE DIET

A healthy diet for everyone, including those with celiac disease, should include a range of nutrients from a variety of foods. Table 1.1 summarizes the minimum recommendations for adults of cereals, vegetables, fruit, dairy, and meat and meat alternatives. These foods should form the basis of our daily diet. Choose the number of servings you need according to your level of activity and your body size. If you are fairly inactive and/or have a small to average body size, choose the lower amount. If you are active and/or have an average to large body size, choose the higher number of servings. If you prefer a diet based on breads and cereals, choose the servings in the unshaded area; however, if you prefer a diet that includes a variety from all food groups, then choose those in the shaded area.

	Servings Daily		
Food Group	Women*	Men*	Serving Size
Cereals	4–9	6–12	2 slices gluten-free bread—2 ounces (60 grams)
	4–6	5–7	$1^3/_4$ cups gluten-free cereal—$2^3/_4$ oz (50 g)
Vegetables	5	5	$^2/_3$ cup cooked vegetables—$2^1/_2$ oz (75 g)
	4–7	6–8	$1^1/_3$ cups salad
Fruit	2	2	1 medium piece
	2–3	3–4	$1^1/_3$ cups diced pieces
Dairy	2	2	8 fl oz (250 ml) milk
	2–4	2–3	$1^1/_2$ oz (40 g) (2 slices) cheese
			7 oz (200 g) (1 container) yogurt
Meat and meat alternatives	1	1	2–$3^1/_2$ oz (65–100 g) cooked meat or chicken
	1–$1^1/_2$	$1^1/_2$–2	$2^1/_2$–4 oz (80–120 g) cooked fish
			2 eggs
			$^2/_3$ cup cooked (dried) peas, beans, or lentils

TABLE 1.1. DAILY MINIMUM SERVING RECOMMENDATIONS ACCORDING TO FOOD GROUP

*19–60 years old

The recommendations in this table are based on the Australian Guide to Healthy Eating (Commonwealth Department of Health and Family Services, 1998).

NUTRIENTS AT RISK ON A GLUTEN-FREE DIET

There are some nutrients that may be limited on a gluten-free diet. For this reason a gluten-free diet should not be entered into lightly, and should only be commenced after confirmation of the diagnosis of celiac disease by a doctor. Calcium, iron, zinc, folic acid (also called folate), and fiber need special consideration on a gluten-free diet. Nutrient deficiencies may occur as a result of the removal of cereals containing gluten, or because of poor nutrient absorption.

Calcium

Osteoporosis is a common complication occurring in celiac disease. Malabsorption of calcium and poor calcium intake are often responsible and contribute to reduced bone mineral density in celiac disease (D. Robertson, "Osteoporosis in Coeliac Disease," *The Australian Coeliac* 8; 3 [1997]: 8). Calcium-rich foods should be included in the diet daily. Good sources of calcium include milk and dairy foods, salmon (including bones), almonds, and unhulled sesame seeds.

Iron

Most of the damage that gluten causes to the gut occurs in the small intestine where iron is absorbed. As a result, iron deficiency is common in those with newly diagnosed celiac disease. Iron is essential in the diet to carry oxygen in the blood. The best sources of iron are animal foods, particularly red meat. Our bodies are able to use the iron in animal foods more readily than in vegetable or cereal foods. Having a food containing vitamin C, such as tomato, orange juice, parsley, or red and green peppers, when having iron-rich vegetable and cereal foods, will increase absorption of iron.

Zinc

Zinc plays a variety of roles in the body, particularly in wound healing, growth, and vision. Cereal foods are a good source of zinc. Zinc intake may be reduced by removing many cereals from the diet. It is important to replace gluten-containing cereals with gluten-free cereals, and regularly include other good sources of zinc such as oysters, meat, chicken, brown rice, beans, eggs, and dairy products.

Folic Acid

Folic acid (or folate) is needed by several enzyme systems in the body and is particularly important during pregnancy. Women who are pregnant or planning pregnancy should discuss taking a folate supplement with their doctor or dietitian. A deficiency of folate can result in anemia. It is not uncommon for someone with newly diagnosed celiac disease to be deficient in folate, due to poor absorption of this nutrient. Good sources of folate include vegetables such as asparagus, spinach, and broccoli, whole-grain bread (gluten-free), nuts, and fresh fruits, especially avocado, bananas, oranges, and cantaloupe.

Fiber

Fruits, vegetables, breads, and cereals (particularly the whole-grain varieties) are the best sources of fiber. High-fiber foods stay in the stomach longer, resulting in an extended feeling of fullness. High-fiber diets also produce softer, bulkier stools and are important in preventing constipation. Many of the best cereal sources of fiber, such as whole-wheat breads and cereals, must be excluded on a gluten-free diet. For adequate fiber it is important to have plenty of fruits and vegetables, legumes such as chickpeas and kidney beans, gluten-free cereals, gluten-free pasta, gluten-free bread, and grains such as rice and corn. The USDA's recommended daily intake of fiber is 38 grams for men aged nineteen to fifty, and 25 grams for women in the same age category. A more advisable intake may be 35–45 grams (3–4 ounces) per day.

TABLE 1.2. GLUTEN-FREE FIBER COUNTER

Food	Serving Size	Grams of Dietary Fiber per Serving
Apples (with skin)	1 medium (5 oz [150 g])	3.0
Apricots (dried)	6 small halves (1 oz [25 g])	2.5
Baked beans	1$\frac{1}{3}$ cups (7 oz [220 g])	10.0
Banana	1 small	3.0
Bean mix (canned) (three-bean mix)	1$\frac{1}{3}$ cups (6 oz [185 g])	11.5
Bread (gluten-free)	1 slice (average)	1.0–2.0
Broccoli	1 large serving (3$\frac{1}{2}$ oz [100 g])	4.0
Cabbage	$\frac{2}{3}$ cup	1.5

Food	Serving Size	Grams of Dietary Fiber per Serving
Carrots (cooked)	$2/_3$ cup (2 oz [70 g])	3.0
Lentils (dry)	$2/_3$ cup ($3^1/_2$ oz [100 g])	9.0
Lentils (cooked)	$1^1/_3$ cups (6 oz [190 g])	6.5
Muesli (gluten-free)	$1^1/_2$ oz (50 g)	5.0
Orange	1 medium	4.0
Peanuts	$1^1/_2$ oz (50 g)	4.0
Peanut butter	1 tablespoon ($3/_4$ oz [20 g])	2.0
Polenta (dry)	2 oz (60 g)	2.0
Potatoes (cooked)	1 medium	2.0
Pumpkin (cooked)	1 piece (3 oz [85 g])	1.5
Rice, brown (cooked)	$1^1/_3$ cups (5 oz [160 g])	3.0
Rice cakes	2	0.5
Rice, white (cooked)	$1^1/_3$ cups (5 oz [175 g])	1.5
Sultanas (golden raisins)	1 tablespoon	1.0
Sweet corn	$2/_3$ cup	2.0

Source: Rosemary Stanton, "Fat and Fibre Counter" in Carolyn O'Gorman, "Fibre for Gluten Free Diet," The Australian Coeliac (1998) Vol. 9; No. 3; pp. 22–23.

WHY ARE THE RECIPES IN THIS BOOK SO GOOD?

The recipes in *Gluten-Free Cooking* can help you to plan healthy food choices and choose foods to help manage celiac disease better. They contain nutrients such as fiber, calcium, iron, zinc, and folate, which are particularly important in celiac disease. They are well balanced and nutritious but most of all they taste delicious!

2.

Dietary Principles

NOT ALL AMERICANS ARE FOLLOWING sound dietary practices. Sound dietary guidelines are an important part of any dietary program. Eating nutritious foods and following healthy lifestyle patterns help promote good health. For sound nutritional practices we should follow these guidelines.

- Enjoy a wide variety of nutritious foods. We need to eat plenty of vegetables and fruits and not forget to include legumes.

- We need plenty of gluten-free meals, and include some gluten-free breads, rice, gluten-free pasta, and gluten-free noodles.

- We should include some lean meat, fish, poultry, and/or alternatives.

- Reduced-fat varieties of milk, yogurts, cheese, and/or alternatives should be included.

- We should drink plenty of water.

- We should take care to:
  - Limit saturated fat and have a moderate total fat intake; choose foods low in salt; limit our alcohol intake if we do choose to drink alcohol, and consume only moderate amounts of sugar and foods containing added sugars.
  - Prevent weight gain: we should be physically active and eat according to our energy needs.

- We should care for our food and prepare and store it safely.

- We should encourage and support breast-feeding.

- A knowledge of the glycemic index of food is helpful for those who require a gluten-free diet and need to watch their blood glucose levels.

The individual with celiac disease is best advised to eat a wide variety of gluten-free foods. They need to maintain an adequate intake of fiber, and nutrients including zinc, iron, and calcium. Sensible eating habits and exercise can help in maintaining a healthy weight. Use the recipes in this book to plan more enjoyable, varied gluten-free meals.

BALANCED GLUTEN-FREE MEALS

An individualized meal plan is best prepared with the guidance of an accredited dietitian practicing in the area of celiac disease. Our meals and snacks should be eaten in a relaxed atmosphere, catered to personal tastes, and be suitable for a gluten-free diet. Regular physical activity and plenty of rest should ensure overall well-being.

GLUTEN-FREE SAMPLE MEAL PLAN

Following is a sample meal plan with meal and snack options.

Breakfast

- Fruit or fruit juice (for vitamin C and fiber)
- Corn or rice cereal (gluten-free) with milk or calcium-fortified soy drink (gluten-free)
- High-fiber, gluten-free toast with a spread of butter/margarine and jam/honey/peanut butter
- Tea, coffee, herbal tea, coffee substitute (gluten-free), milk, fortified soy drink (gluten-free), or water

Lunch (or evening meal)

- Choose fish, lean meat, lean poultry, egg, cheese, or peanut butter with salads and/or cooked vegetables
- High-fiber (gluten-free) bread with a spread of butter/margarine/cream cheese or gluten-free chutney or mustard
- Fruit (fresh or tinned) or gluten-free yogurt
- Tea, coffee, herbal tea, coffee substitute (gluten-free), milk, fortified soy drink (gluten-free), fresh fruit juice (no added sugar), or water

Main Meal (lunch or evening meal)

- Stir-fried beef or chicken flavored with a gluten-free soy sauce, garlic, and grated ginger

- Vegetables and rice or rice vermicelli

- Chopped fruit and gluten-free yogurt or custard

- Tea, coffee, herbal tea, coffee substitute (gluten-free), milk, fortified soy drink (gluten-free), fresh fruit juice (no added sugar), or water

Mid-Morning, Mid-Afternoon, and Evening Snacks

- Fresh fruit

- Gluten-free crackers with cheese

- Healthy muffins (gluten-free)

- Tea, coffee, herbal tea, coffee substitute (gluten-free), milk, fortified soy drink (gluten-free), fresh fruit juice (no added sugar), or water

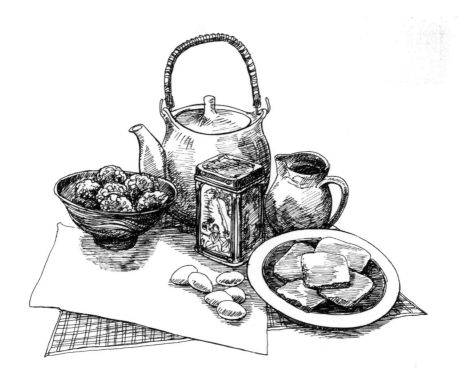

3.

Celiac Disease
and Gluten-Free Diets

CELIAC DISEASE IS A CONDITION in which the lining of the small bowel (intestine) is damaged when it is exposed to gluten. Gluten is the main protein found in the cereal grains wheat, oats, barley, rye, and triticale. Even small amounts of gluten cause damage to the small bowel. There are many obvious foods such as bread, cakes, cereals, and cookies that contain gluten. There are also many foods and ingredients that are less obvious such as sausages, corn flour (of wheat origin) sauces, gravies, and malt vinegar.

You may ask the question "Why did I develop celiac disease?" The answer is unknown. Both genetic and environmental factors play important roles in celiac disease. Common symptoms can include anemia, bloating, chronic diarrhea, flatulence, constipation, stomach pain, vomiting, and/or weight loss. Children may experience growth retardation.

Normally, food passes from the stomach into the small intestine (the first part of this is called the duodenum) where it is gradually digested and absorbed into the system. Leftover material passes into the large intestine (colon), and is eventually expelled. The small intestine is a long tube lined with folds called "villi." These villi project into the intestine like "fingers" and increase the surface area. In celiac disease these villi are damaged by gluten and the mucosa becomes "flat" and inflamed so that the area available for absorption is much reduced. Because of this, unabsorbed food passes down to the large intestine and out in the bowel motions. A lot of this food is fermented and made rotten by bacteria living in the large intestine. The abdomen may be "bloated" by the gases produced by undigested food. Nutrient and vitamin deficiencies can result from poor absorption of food.

The only treatment for celiac disease is a gluten-free diet. Once this is established the mucosa steadily return to normal and digestion and absorption of food is greatly improved. The severity of the symptoms in this disease vary widely. Some children are greatly affected early in life following the introduction of gluten-containing cereals while others are not affected until much later. Many of those diagnosed are adults and of these, a fairly high percentage are over the age of forty. A small bowel biopsy prior to the commencement of a gluten-free diet is required to establish the diagnosis and a lifelong avoidance of gluten in the diet is necessary.

It must be noted that there are people in the community who do not have celiac disease but have an intolerance to gluten. These people will find that they can experience improvement in their digestive system and general health if they do not eat foods that contain gluten.

TESTING FOR CELIAC DISEASE

Celiac disease is diagnosed by a small bowel biopsy that is carried out by a gastroenterologist. It is possible for other conditions to mimic celiac disease and only this special test can diagnose the condition. The flattening of the small bowel villi is indicative of celiac disease. This test should be performed before the commencement of a gluten-free diet. After the onset of a gluten-free diet the damaged lining of the intestine can repair itself. Some doctors will use a blood test as a screening tool before recommending a biopsy.

Celiac disease is a lifelong dietary intolerance to gluten. The gluten-free diet is a treatment, not a cure. This diet is a major change that requires a positive attitude and some time and effort in the initial stages. It is important to exclude all forms of gluten. If a gluten-free diet is not maintained damage to the lining of the small bowel (intestine) can be such that food is not absorbed properly. Many celiacs may be tempted to rely on gut symptoms to determine whether a doubtful food is safe. This is an inaccurate and dangerous practice as symptoms may not appear immediately after eating a food, but can have long-term impacts on the nutritional status and can increase the risk of bowel cancer. Even small amounts of gluten may affect people with celiac disease and result in weight loss, chronic diarrhea, mouth ulcerations, constipation, and other symptoms.

WHEN TO EXPECT RELIEF
FROM YOUR GLUTEN-FREE DIET

Some people find relief from their symptoms within days of excluding gluten from their diet. Others find it may take months before an appreciable improvement can be noticed. Some patients will get further relief over a period of one or two years. Everyone is an individual. If symptoms fail to improve or become worse it is possible that gluten is being consumed in hidden forms. Common mistakes are the inclusion of thickeners, malt, or one inconspicuous source is the Communion host. Remember that the ingestion of a Communion host once a week may be enough to cause bowel damage with or without significant symptoms.

RESOURCES AND LINKS TO CELIAC SOCIETIES

Celiac.com

Celiac.com is a website that provides resources and information for people on gluten-free diets due to celiac disease, gluten intolerance, dermatitis herpetiformis, wheat allergy, or other health reasons. It includes listings of celiac societies and local support groups, important food ingredient information, as well as links to newsletters, magazines, and articles.

Website: http://www.celiac.com

CELIAC (Celiac/Coeliac Wheat/Gluten-Free List)

The CELIAC listserve is an open, unmoderated discussion for those interested in celiac disease, dermatitis herpetiformis, gluten intolerance, wheat allergy, and coincident intolerances, such as casein or lactose intolerance. Included on the website are listings of local support groups.

Websites: http://www.enabling.org/ia/celiac/groups/groupsus.html
http://www.enabling.org/ia/celiac/index.html#support

Celiac Disease Foundation (CDF)

CDF is a national celiac disease support group that provides information and assistance to people affected by celiac disease/dermatitis herpetiformis (CD/DH). The Celiac Disease Foundation publishes *Guidelines for a Gluten-Free Lifestyle,* which includes information on FDA labeling laws and is free for members.

Contact: Celiac Disease Foundation
             13251 Ventura Blvd., #1
             Studio City, CA 91604
             (818) 990-2354 • http://www.celiac.org

Celiac Sprue Association (CSA)

CSA is a nonprofit celiac support group in the United States, with over 100 chapters and 60 resource units across the country, and over 10,000 members worldwide.

Contact: Celiac Sprue Association
             P.O. Box 31700
             Omaha, NE 68131-0700
             (877) CSA-4-CSA (toll-free) • http://www.csaceliacs.org

The Gluten-Free Mall

This online shopping center, an offshoot of celiac.com, offers a selection of gluten-free, wheat-free, casein-free, and other allergy-related health foods and special dietary products.

Website: http://www.glutenfreemall.com

GlutenSmart

This online store sells gluten-free food products and publishes a newsletter.

Website: http://www.glutensmart.com

TABLE 3.1. A HANDY FOOD LIST FOR CELIACS		
Food	Foods Allowed	Foods to Avoid
Alcohol	Distilled alcoholic drinks, wines, and fortified wines. Port, sherry, brandy, cognac, rum, liqueurs, champagne. Remember if you drink alcohol, limit your intake.	Ale, stout, beer, lager. Some alcoholic drinks may contain gluten ingredients.
Alfalfa seeds	Gluten-free.	
Almond meal	Can be used in conjunction with other gluten-free flours.	
Amaranth	Gluten-free flour that is best used in combination with other flours in gluten-free cooking.	

Arrowroot	A starch made from the tuber of a West Indian plant that is gluten-free. It is a finer starch than corn flour and can be used in place of corn flour as a thickener or in cake and cookie making.	
Baby rice cereal	Can be used with other gluten-free flours in baking.	
Baking powder	Only those with gluten-free ingredients.	Read labels carefully as some baking powder may contain ingredients that are not gluten-free.
Barbecue chicken	Chickens cooked without stuffing, seasoning, or marinades.	Chicken cooked with bread stuffing that is not gluten-free. The seasoning mix used to coat some cooked chickens may not be gluten-free.
Barley		Must not be eaten.
Battered foods	Homemade gluten-free batter.	Not allowed when the batter is made from gluten flours.
Beans	Soy beans, kidney beans, cannellini beans, borlotti beans, garbanzo beans, black-eyed peas, navy beans, mung beans, lentils. Beans are an excellent source of fiber for the diet.	Processed beans may be thickened with gluten-containing ingredients and should be checked.
Besan	This is chickpea flour and is suitable in a gluten-free diet.	
Beverages	Coffee, tea, plain cocoa, soft drinks (no barley), mineral water. Some drinking chocolates are suitable.	Coffee substitutes that contain wheat or barley. Some drinking chocolates and malted drinks. Additives in herbal and instant teas may contain gluten. Barley water. Nondairy whitener. Read labels carefully to check for ingredients that may contain gluten.
Bran	Soy bran or rice bran.	Wheat bran, oat bran, and wheat germ.
Bread	Gluten-free breads. Choose high-fiber breads made from a variety of gluten-free cereals. Commercial gluten-free bread mixes. Gluten-free bread crumbs.	Commercial breads (unless marked gluten-free), croissants, crispbreads, bread crumbs, bread seasonings (watch stuffings in meats and prepared chickens), crumpets, muffins. Watch coating on foods.
Breakfast cereals	Rice and corn cereals (check for added malt and malt extract as these are barley products and are not gluten-free). Some gluten-free cornflakes are available. Homemade and commercial gluten-free muesli, using allowed ingredients. Choose high-fiber breakfast cereals with no added sugar if possible.	Muesli, semolina, triticale, wheat bran, wheat germ, wheatmeal, oat bran, oatmeal, and rolled oats.

Buckwheat	Buckwheat is the fruit of an herbaceous plant (*Fagopyrum esculentum*). It does not contain gluten and can be used as kernels or as flour in cooking.	
Butter and margarine	Butter and margarine are gluten-free. Limit added fats if necessary on a low-fat, weight-reduction diet.	Those following a gluten-free diet should watch for contamination of margarine/butter during shared use. It is best to use a separate container.
Buttermilk	Cultured buttermilk.	
Cakes	Gluten-free mixes and cakes are available.	Cakes, cookies, pastries (unless made with gluten-free ingredients). For a healthy diet limit high-fat and high-sugar varieties.
Caramel color	If made in North America it is likely to be gluten-free.	
Cassava	Cassava is the tuber of the cassava plant and is part of the staple diet in many tropical countries. Tapioca is also prepared from the cassava tuber.	
Cheese	Block and cheddar cheese (choose low-fat, low-salt as desired), cottage cheese, ricotta cheese, light cream cheese (such as Philadelphia, Organic Valley, or Horizon brands).	Read labels carefully as processed cheeses, cheese pastes, cheese flavor, and spreads may contain gluten.
Chicken	Fresh and frozen plain varieties. Remove all skin and fat before use for healthy eating.	Prepared whole chickens with prepared stuffing, coating, processed chicken products.
Chickpeas	Chickpea flour is also known as besan.	
Chocolate	Plain chocolate. (Limit intake on a low-fat diet.)	Refer to ingredient information as some chocolate fillings may contain gluten.
Chutney	Those made from gluten-free ingredients.	Check labels carefully as some commercial varieties may contain gluten ingredients.
Coconut	Gluten-free.	
Coffee	Coffee grounds. Instant and drip coffee.	Coffee substitutes, coffee mixes, coffee milk flavorings. Read labels carefully as some products may contain gluten ingredients. Barley is often used in coffee substitutes.
Commercial bread mixes	Gluten-free bread mixes are allowed.	Ordinary bread mixes are not allowed.
Cookies and crackers	Rice cookies, rice crackers, and rice crispbreads, and those cookies and crackers marked gluten-free.	Commercial cookies and crackers (unless marked gluten-free). Not all rice crackers are gluten-free and may include unsuitable ingredients that contain gluten, for example, soy sauce.

Corn	This is allowed in all forms, for example, polenta (cornmeal) and maize meal.	
Corn chips	Plain corn chips.	Flavored corn chips and similar products may have added gluten-containing ingredients.
Corned beef	Gluten-free unless gluten ingredients are added during cooking.	Corned beef cooked in malt vinegar is not gluten-free.
Cornflakes	There are gluten-free varieties available. Check for addition of malt and malt extract as these are barley products and are not gluten-free.	Check labels carefully as some varieties may contain gluten ingredients.
Corn flour	Corn flour from maize.	Wheaten corn flour.
Cream	Fresh or canned varieties are gluten-free. (Limit intake on a low-fat diet.)	Artificial cream products may not be gluten-free.
Curry	Curry spices are gluten-free, but check other ingredients.	Read labels carefully as some commercial varieties may contain gluten products.
Custard	Maize corn flour custard powder. Prepared custards made from gluten-free ingredients.	Check labels carefully as some commercial varieties may contain gluten ingredients.
Deli meats	Gluten-free varieties are available—check ingredients.	Processed meats may contain gluten ingredients. Read labels carefully and always check ingredients with deli staff before purchasing.
Eggs	Include in diet as desired.	
Fish	Plain fresh varieties. Grill or microwave, or fry in a nonstick pan with a little cooking spray.	Fish fingers. Read labels carefully on tinned fish, for example, sardines in sauce. Be careful as some restaurants dust grilled fish with flour. Fish crumbed in bread crumbs that are not gluten-free.
Flour	Lentil, pea, potato, rice, taro, soy. Commercial gluten-free flours.	Wheat, rye, oaten, barley, triticale.
Fondant	Gluten-free varieties available—check ingredients.	Read labels carefully as some fondant contains gluten ingredients.
Fruit	Fresh, frozen, canned, juices.	Commercial fruit pie fillings may be thickened with ingredients that are not gluten-free.
Gelatin	Gluten-free.	
Glucose syrup	Gluten-free even if derived from wheat.	
Golden syrup	Gluten-free.	
Gravy thickeners	Gluten-free gravy mixes.	Check all labels carefully. Avoid gravy when eating out unless you know that it is gluten-free.

Guar gum	Gluten-free.	
Ham	Gluten-free varieties are available—check ingredients.	Read labels carefully or ask deli staff as some ham may contain gluten ingredients.
Herbs and spices	Fresh herbs.	Some herb and spice mixes may contain gluten ingredients.
Honey	Gluten-free.	
Hydrolyzed vegetable protein (HPV)	HVP from maize or soy is gluten-free. If the source is unidentified it is gluten-free.	May contain gluten.
Ice cream	A number of varieties made from gluten-free ingredients are available.	Check labels for those containing ingredients that are not gluten-free, for example, cookie crumbs and ice-cream cones.
Icing sugar	Pure icing sugar.	Icing sugar mixture may contain ingredients that are not gluten-free.
Jam	Gluten-free.	Watch for contamination with gluten bread crumbs if sharing products.
Legumes	Legumes are the edible seeds and/or pods of the pulse family (peas, beans, and lentils). Legumes add fiber to the diet and are gluten-free.	
Lentils	Lentils are a variety of legume.	
Licorice	Licorice extract is gluten-free.	Read labels carefully as it may contain gluten ingredients.
LSA	Initials stand for linseed, sunflower, and almond. Adds nutritional value to products like muffins and bread.	
Lupins	Gluten-free.	
Malt	Malt from rice or other gluten-free ingredients.	Malt and malt extracts.
Maltodextrin	Maltodextrins are used in commercial products for sweetening and stabilizing. Maltodextrin from maize is gluten-free. If the source is unidentified it is gluten-free.	Maltodextrin made from wheat may not be gluten-free.
Maple syrup	Gluten-free.	
Marinades	Those made from gluten-free ingredients.	Read labels carefully as some may contain gluten ingredients.
Marzipan	Those made from gluten-free ingredients.	Read labels carefully as some may contain gluten ingredients.

Mayonnaise	Those made from gluten-free ingredients.	Read labels carefully as some have malt vinegar and gluten ingredients.
Meat	Plain lean meats with no additives.	Read labels carefully or ask deli staff as processed meats may contain gluten ingredients.
Milk	Fresh, UHT (ultra-high temperature), evaporated, condensed, powdered.	Malted milk. Read labels carefully on flavored milks as some may contain gluten ingredients.
Millet	Gluten-free.	
Monosodium glutamate	MSG and other glutamates are gluten-free.	
Mustard	Seed varieties.	Check labels of powdered and prepared varieties carefully.
Nuts	All unflavored and salted varieties.	Dry roasted nuts may be dusted with flour and may not be gluten-free.
Oats		Contain gluten.
Oils	As desired. Limit intake on a low-fat diet.	
Olives	As desired.	
Pasta	Pasta from soy, rice, corn, and other gluten-free sources can be eaten. There is now a wide range of gluten-free pasta on the market.	Wheat flour pasta, such as macaroni or noodles.
Pastes	Those made from gluten-free ingredients.	Read labels carefully as some may contain gluten ingredients.
Peanut butter	As desired. Freshly processed varieties are a good choice.	Read labels carefully as some peanut butter may contain gluten ingredients, for example, maltodextrin made from wheat.
Pickles and chutney	Homemade varieties are best, made without malt vinegar.	Read labels carefully as some may contain gluten ingredients.
Polenta	Polenta is the Italian name for cornmeal. It is excellent for adding gluten-free fiber to the diet.	
Popcorn	Gluten-free.	Read labels carefully as some added flavors may contain gluten ingredients.
Poppy seeds	Gluten-free.	
Potato chips	Plain varieties that do not contain wheat.	Read labels carefully as some added flavors may contain gluten ingredients
Potato wedges	Homemade from gluten-free ingredients.	Commercial varieties contain gluten ingredients.

Psyllium	A fiber food from the psyllium plant.	
Pumpkin seeds	Gluten-free.	
Quinoa	A high-protein grain resembling millet.	
Rice	All rice is gluten-free. Basmati is good for those interested in watching the GI (glycemic index) factor in their food intake.	Read labels carefully as some prepared commercial rice products may contain gluten ingredients.
Rice bran	Adds excellent fiber to a gluten-free diet.	
Rice flour	Brown or white rice flour is suitable for gluten-free cooking.	
Rye		Contains gluten—not allowed.
Sago	Gluten-free.	
Salami	Gluten-free varieties are available—check ingredients.	Read labels carefully as some varieties may contain gluten ingredients.
Sauces	Gluten-free varieties are available—check ingredients.	Read labels carefully as some varieties may contain gluten ingredients.
Sausages	Gluten-free varieties are available—check ingredients.	Read labels carefully as some varieties may contain gluten ingredients.
Semolina		Not allowed as this is made from wheaten flour.
Sesame seeds	Gluten-free.	
Sorghum	Gluten-free grain that can be made into flour.	
Soups	Homemade gluten-free soups made with gluten-free stock cubes. Some commercial soups are gluten-free.	Read labels carefully as some may contain gluten ingredients, such as barley and noodle thickeners made from wheat.
Sourdough		Not gluten-free.
Soy	Use as beans, grits, flakes, or flour.	Read labels carefully as some soy sauces may contain gluten ingredients.
Soy sauce	Gluten-free varieties are available—check ingredients.	Read labels carefully as some brands contain gluten ingredients.
Spelt (flour)		Not gluten-free.
Starch	Corn, tapioca, maize, potato. Those that are unidentified are gluten-free.	Those from wheat.
Stock	Gluten-free varieties are available—check ingredients.	Check labels carefully as some stock cubes, stock powders, and UHT stock may contain ingredients that are not gluten-free.

Sugar	Gluten-free.	
Sunflower seeds	Gluten-free.	
Sushi	Most sushi is gluten-free—check ingredients.	Read labels carefully or check at the deli, as some added ingredients may not be gluten-free, for example, soy sauce.
Tabouli		Contains cracked wheat.
Taco shells	Most commercial shells are gluten-free.	Read labels carefully as some may contain gluten ingredients.
Tamari	Gluten-free varieties are available— check ingredients.	Read labels carefully as some tamari may contain gluten ingredients.
Tapioca	Gluten-free.	
Tea	Tea leaves and tea bags.	Read labels carefully as some instant tea and tea substitutes may contain gluten ingredients.
Thickeners	Corn, tapioca, maize, potato. Those that are unidentified are gluten-free.	Those made with wheat or other grains that contain gluten.
Triticale		Not allowed as this is a hybrid of wheat and rye.
Vanilla	Gluten-free in all forms, vanilla extract and vanilla essence.	
Vegetables	Fresh, frozen, canned, dried, and juices.	Read labels carefully as some vegetable products may contain gluten ingredients.
Vinegar	White distilled vinegar, balsamic vinegar, and other vinegars without malt.	Malt vinegar.
Water chestnuts	Gluten-free.	
Wheat		Not gluten-free.
Worcestershire sauce	Limited gluten-free varieties available— check ingredients.	Most brands contain wheat or gluten sources.
Yeast	Dehydrated and compressed yeast can be purchased at some supermarkets and health food stores. It is suitable to use in gluten-free bread making.	Brewers yeast is not gluten-free.
Yeast extract	Gluten-free yeast extracts are available.	Extracts containing malt should not be consumed.
Yogurt	Gluten-free varieties are available— check ingredients.	Read labels carefully as some commercial varieties may contain gluten ingredients.

Note: Manufacturers do change the composition of food products. Therefore, those requiring a gluten-free diet must be aware that food products are subject to change. It is necessary to continually check ingredients on all products on a frequent basis to ensure all products consumed are gluten-free.

PART II
Recipes

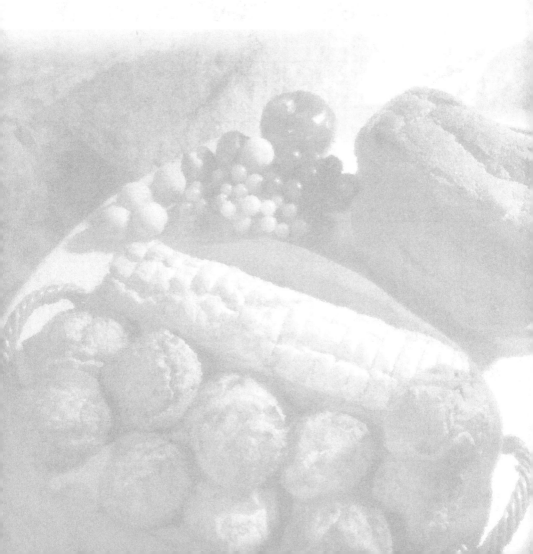

MEASUREMENTS AND CONVERSION TABLES

Measurements in this book are made using U.S. standard unit cup and spoon measures. All spoon measurements are level spoonfuls, unless otherwise stated.

A kitchen scale is necessary for some of the recipes in which dry ingredients such as flour and sugar are listed by weight (ounces and/or pounds). Using a scale allows for more precise measurement, which is particularly important in making bread and some other baked goods.

Commonly Accepted Metric Conversions Used in Cookery

WEIGHT	
Avoirdupois (U.S.)	Metric
$\frac{1}{2}$ ounce	15 grams
1 ounce	30 grams
2 ounces	60 grams
3 ounces	90 grams
4 ounces ($\frac{1}{4}$ pound)	110 grams
5 ounces	140 grams
6 ounces	170 grams
7 ounces	200 grams
8 ounces ($\frac{1}{2}$ pound)	230 grams
9 ounces	280 grams
10 ounces	315 grams
11 ounces	345 grams
12 ounces ($\frac{3}{4}$ pound)	375 grams
13 ounces	410 grams
14 ounces	440 grams
15 ounces	470 grams
16 ounces (1 pound)	500 grams (0.5 kilogram)
24 ounces ($1\frac{1}{2}$ pounds)	750 grams
32 ounces (2 pounds)	1,000 grams (1 kilogram)
3 pounds	1,500 grams (1.5 kilograms)
4 pounds	2,000 grams (2 kilograms)

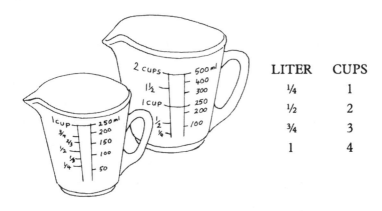

LITER	CUPS	MLS
¼	1	250
½	2	500
¾	3	750
1	4	1000

VOLUME	
Imperial (U.S.)	Metric
1 fluid ounce	30 milliliters
3 fluid ounces	100 milliliters
5 fluid ounces	150 milliliters
8 fluid ounces (¹/₂ pint or 1 cup)	250 milliliters
10 fluid ounces	300 milliliters
16 fluid ounces (1 pint)	500 milliliters
20 fluid ounces	600 milliliters

1 tablespoon 20 ml

1 teaspoon 5 ml

½ teaspoon 2.5 ml

¼ teaspoon 1.25 ml

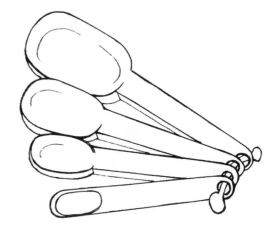

Oven Temperatures

It is very difficult to advise on exact oven temperatures. Different makes of stoves give different results at the same temperature setting. You are the best judge of the heat settings of your own stove for the particular product you are cooking. The cooking time for a product can vary greatly between different kinds of stoves. Fan-forced ovens in the newer stoves have reduced cooking times considerably. Also, many of the foods in this book can be successfully prepared in a microwave oven. In this case, cooking times will be greatly reduced, and further variations in cooking time are possible depending on the heat setting chosen. The table "Oven Temperatures" should be a helpful guide to making appropriate selections.

OVEN TEMPERATURES				
	Electricity		Gas	
	Fahrenheit	Celsius	Fahrenheit	Celsius
Very slow	250	120	250	120
Slow	300	150	275–300	140–150
Moderately slow	325–350	160–180	325	160
Moderate	375–400	190–200	350	180
Moderately hot	425–450	220–230	375	190
Hot	475–500	250–260	400–450	200–230
Very hot	525–550	270–290	475–500	250–260

Microwave Oven Cooking Times

A 900 watt microwave oven has been used when making recipes in this book. Microwave cooking times will vary with different wattage ovens, type of container, temperature and volume of ingredients, and so on. There is no way to accurately predict cooking times. A good rule to remember is always to undercook rather than overcook.

Abbreviations

fl oz = fluid ounce	lb = pound	oz = ounce
g = gram	mg = milligram	pt = pint

4.

Breakfast

Buckwheat Pancakes, 30

Flapjacks, 31

Muesli, 32

Pancakes with Raspberry Spread, 33

Rice and Raisin Porridge, 35

Ricotta Pancakes, 36

Vegetable-Rice Patties, 37

BUCKWHEAT PANCAKES

These pancakes are made with rice flour and buckwheat flour.

PREPARATION TIME: 20 minutes • COOKING TIME: 15 minutes

YIELD: Approximately 20 pancakes

$^2/_3$ cup brown rice flour

2 cups buckwheat flour

2 teaspoons gluten-free baking powder

$^1/_2$ teaspoon baking soda

1 tablespoon finely granulated white sugar

2 tablespoons salt-reduced monounsaturated margarine

$2^1/_3$ cups cultured buttermilk

$^1/_2$ teaspoon vanilla extract

A little oil to grease electric skillet

1. Sift brown rice flour, buckwheat flour, baking powder, and baking soda into a medium-sized mixing bowl. Stir in sugar.

2. Place margarine into a small saucepan. Melt over a low heat.

OR Place margarine into a small microwave-safe bowl. Microwave on high for 30 seconds or until margarine is melted.

3. Stir buttermilk and vanilla into melted margarine.

4. Pour liquid into dry ingredients and mix to a thick batter consistency.

5. Heat an electric skillet to 340°F. Lightly oil skillet.

6. Place tablespoons of mixture into heated skillet.

7. Cook on one side until mixture is set on the surface. Turn and cook on reverse side until golden brown and cooked.

8. Place plastic wrap over a fine wire rack. When cooked, remove pancakes from skillet and place onto wire rack. Cover with plastic wrap to prevent drying out.

FLAPJACKS

These delicious flapjacks will tempt any palate.

PREPARATION TIME: 20 minutes • COOKING TIME: 15 minutes
YIELD: Approximately 20 flapjacks

$1\frac{1}{3}$ cups white rice flour

$\frac{2}{3}$ cup buckwheat flour

2 teaspoons gluten-free baking powder

1 teaspoon baking soda

$\frac{1}{2}$ cup finely granulated white sugar

4 tablespoons salt-reduced monounsaturated margarine

1 egg

$1\frac{2}{3}$ cups cultured buttermilk

$\frac{1}{4}$ teaspoon vanilla extract

A little oil to grease electric skillet

1. Sift rice flour, buckwheat flour, baking powder, and baking soda into a medium-sized mixing bowl. Stir in sugar.

2. Place margarine into a small saucepan. Melt over a low heat.

OR Place margarine into a microwave-safe bowl. Microwave on high for 30 seconds or until margarine is melted.

3. Break egg into a small bowl and beat well. Stir melted margarine, buttermilk, and vanilla into egg.

4. Pour liquid into dry ingredients and mix to a thick batter consistency, adding a little more buttermilk if necessary.

5. Heat an electric skillet to 340°F. Lightly oil skillet.

6. Place tablespoons of mixture into heated skillet.

7. Cook on one side until mixture is set on the surface. Turn and cook on reverse side until golden brown and cooked.

8. Place plastic wrap over a fine wire rack. When cooked, remove flapjacks from skillet and place onto wire rack. Cover with plastic wrap to prevent drying out.

MUESLI

*Homemade muesli is very nutritious. You can put your own choice of
ingredients into your muesli. This is a good combination of ingredients.
The muesli will be softer to eat if it is soaked overnight with your
favorite addition of low-fat milk, soy drink, or buttermilk.*

PREPARATION TIME: 15 minutes

$5\frac{1}{3}$ cups rolled rice flakes

$1\frac{1}{3}$ cups rice bran

$\frac{2}{3}$ cup toasted coconut
(omit on a low-cholesterol diet)

$\frac{2}{3}$ cup toasted almond flakes

$\frac{2}{3}$ cup sunflower seed kernels

$\frac{2}{3}$ cup natural golden raisins (sultanas)

$\frac{2}{3}$ cup chopped natural raisins

2 tablespoons skim-milk powder

$\frac{2}{3}$ cup chopped dried apricots

1. Mix all the ingredients together.

2. Store in an airtight container until required.

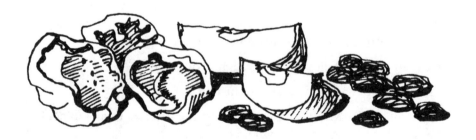

PANCAKES WITH RASPBERRY SPREAD

These pancakes are gluten-free and have no added fat.
They can be served with the delicious raspberry spread recipe
below given to me by my friend Denise.

PANCAKES PREPARATION TIME: 8 minutes • COOKING TIME: 20 minutes
RASPBERRY SPREAD PREPARATION TIME: 5 minutes • COOKING TIME: 7 minutes
YIELD: 12 large pancakes, approximately 3 cups raspberry spread

Pancakes

2 egg whites

$^2/_3$ cup finely granulated white sugar

$^2/_3$ cup milk

1 tablespoon golden syrup (such as Lyle's)

$^1/_2$ teaspoon vanilla extract

2 cups gluten-free self-raising flour

$^1/_2$ teaspoon baking soda

$^2/_3$ cup low-fat natural yogurt

Raspberry Spread

2 teaspoons gelatin

2 tablespoons cold water

2 cups (total) apple and pear juice

14 oz frozen raspberries

Pancakes

1. Place egg whites into a large dry, clean mixing bowl. Beat whites until they hold stiff peaks.

2. Gradually add sugar to egg whites, beating well after each addition.

3. Pour milk into a measuring jug. Pour in golden syrup. Warm milk in the microwave for 30 seconds and stir. Warm for another 30 seconds and stir. Stir in vanilla.

4. Add flour and liquid alternately to the egg mixture, mixing well after each addition.

5. Stir baking soda into yogurt. Stir into mixture. Mixture should be a batter consistency.

6. Heat an electric skillet to 340°F. Spray skillet with cooking spray.

7. Place tablespoons of mixture into skillet.

8. Cook until bubbles appear on the surface. Turn and cook on reverse side until golden brown.

9. Place plastic wrap over a fine wire rack. When cooked, remove pancakes from skillet and place onto wire rack. Cover with plastic wrap to prevent drying out.

Raspberry Spread

1. Place gelatin into a small saucepan. Stir in water. Allow to stand for 2 minutes. Add apple and pear juice. Bring to a boil over a gentle heat.

2. Add raspberries.

3. Bring to a boil and simmer for 7 minutes or until sauce has slightly thickened.

4. Remove from heat and bottle while still hot in warm sterilized jars.

5. When cool, store in the refrigerator. It will keep for approximately two weeks in the refrigerator.

RICE AND RAISIN PORRIDGE

This recipe is easy to prepare and makes an interesting variation for a hot breakfast cereal. For best results it is necessary to soak rice and raisins overnight. This is a good wholesome breakfast for one person.

PREPARATION TIME: 5 minutes • COOKING TIME: 5 minutes
(4 minutes in microwave)
YIELD: 1 serving

⅓ cup brown rice
⅓ cup natural raisins, cut in half
1⅓ cups water, gluten-free soy drink,
or low-fat milk, as desired

1. Place rice into a small microwave-safe bowl.

2. Add raisins and liquid.

3. Cover bowl and allow to soak overnight.

4. The next morning place into a small saucepan and cook until rice is tender and liquid is absorbed (approximately 5 minutes), stirring occasionally.

OR Microwave on high until rice is tender and liquid is absorbed (approximately 4 minutes), stirring occasionally.

5. Serve with honey and sprinkle with cinnamon as desired.

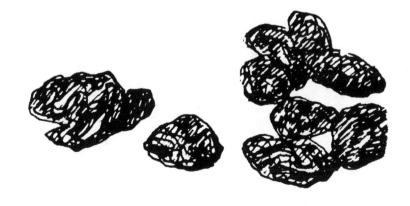

RICOTTA PANCAKES

Ricotta pancakes are great for breakfast.

PREPARATION TIME: 15 minutes • COOKING TIME: 30 minutes
YIELD: Approximately 20 pancakes (3$\frac{1}{2}$" to 4" in diameter)

1$\frac{1}{3}$ cups gluten-free, plain,
all-purpose flour

1 teaspoon gluten-free baking powder

8 oz smooth ricotta

$\frac{2}{3}$ cup low-fat milk

2 eggs, separated

1. Place gluten-free flour, baking powder, ricotta, milk, and egg yolks into an electric blender and blend until smooth.

2. In a separate, clean, dry bowl, beat egg whites until stiff. Lightly fold into mixture in blender.

3. Heat an electric skillet to 340°F. Spray with cooking spray.

4. Use the jug from the blender as a pouring jug and pour small portions of batter into heated skillet.

5. Cook on one side until bubbles appear on surface. Turn and cook on reverse side until golden brown.

6. When cooked, place the pancakes onto a fine wire rack to cool. Place onto a flat plate and cover with plastic wrap to prevent drying.

7. Re-grease pan as necessary for further cooking.

VEGETABLE-RICE PATTIES

PREPARATION TIME: **10 minutes** • COOKING TIME: **15 minutes**
YIELD: **6 servings**

$\frac{2}{3}$ cup basmati rice

1$\frac{1}{3}$ cups boiling water

2$\frac{2}{3}$ cups grated vegetables (of your choice)

1 onion, peeled and finely grated

1 clove garlic, peeled and crushed

2 tablespoons grated parmesan cheese

Salt and pepper, as desired

2 eggs, lightly beaten

$\frac{1}{3}$ cup gluten-free corn flour

3 tablespoons olive oil

1. Place rice into a medium-sized bowl. Pour boiling water over rice. Cook over a gentle heat until rice is soft. Strain and discard any liquid.

2. Add grated vegetables, onion, garlic, and parmesan cheese to rice. Season as desired. Add egg and mix well.

3. Shape into patties approximately $\frac{1}{2}$ inch in thickness.

4. Toss each patty in corn flour.

5. Pour a little olive oil into a large frying pan, or spray pan with cooking spray. Heat over a gentle heat.

6. Increase to a moderate heat. Add patties. Cook for approximately 4 minutes. Turn carefully and cook on reverse side. Patties can be cooked in egg rings if desired. When cooked, carefully remove from pan and drain on absorbent paper.

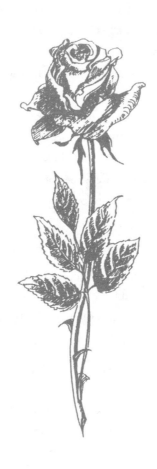

5.

Soups and Starters

Soups
Bell Pepper Soup, 40
Celery and Lentil Soup, 41
Curried Vegetable Soup, 42
Meatball Soup, 43
Tomato Soup, 45

Starters
Baked Avocado with Crab, 46
Baked Omelette Roll, 48
Prawn Aspic Molds, 50
Sardine Dip, 51
Salmon Pâté, 52
Smoked Salmon Sushi, 53

BELL PEPPER SOUP

PREPARATION TIME: $1\frac{1}{2}$ hours
YIELD: **6 servings**

6 medium-sized red bell peppers

$\frac{1}{3}$ cup olive oil

3 cloves garlic, peeled and crushed

3 medium-sized onions,
peeled and cut into $\frac{1}{2}$-inch cubes

2 large potatoes

2 carrots

1 stick celery

1 bay leaf

3 sprigs thyme

3 cups gluten-free stock, as desired

$\frac{1}{4}$ teaspoon chopped chili,
more or less as desired

Salt and pepper, as desired

Sour cream, for serving

Parmesan cheese, for serving

1. Preheat oven to 350°F.

2. Prepare a flat oven tray by spraying with cooking spray.

3. Wash and dry peppers. Brush with a little oil. Place onto prepared tray. Place into a moderate oven and bake for approximately 55 minutes or until just collapsed, taking care to turn during cooking to prevent burning.

4. When pepper is cooked, remove from oven and allow to cool. Remove stalks and seeds. Reserve any cooking juices to add to stock.

5. Heat remaining oil in a nonstick pan. Sauté garlic. Add onion and sauté for 5 minutes or until soft.

6. Peel and cut potatoes and carrots into $\frac{1}{2}$-inch cubes. Place into cold water. Bring to a boil. Boil for 1 minute. Strain and discard water.

7. Add garlic, onions, celery, bay leaf, thyme, and stock. Simmer gently over a low heat until vegetables are soft.

8. Add pepper and any juices to soup. Stir in chili as desired. Bring to a boil and simmer for 5 minutes.

9. Remove from heat. Allow to cool. When cool, remove bay leaf and thyme.

10. Place into the bowl of an electric food blender and blend until smooth (or rub through a sieve). Season as desired.

11. Serve hot with sour cream and freshly grated parmesan cheese.

CELERY AND LENTIL SOUP

Lentils are an excellent addition to a meat-free diet.
They are rich in nutrients and fiber.

PREPARATION TIME: **10 minutes** • COOKING TIME: **1 hour**
YIELD: **6 servings**

$\frac{1}{2}$ bunch celery

8 cups water

2 large potatoes, peeled
and cut into small cubes

1 onion, peeled
and cut into small cubes

8 oz green lentils

2 teaspoons gluten-free
concentrated vegetable stock

1. Wash celery stalks and leaves and cut into small pieces.

2. Place chopped celery and remaining ingredients into a large saucepan.

3. Simmer with lid on until vegetables are soft (approximately 1 hour).

4. Blend in an electric food processor or blender or rub through a sieve or food mill.

5. Reheat to serve.

CURRIED VEGETABLE SOUP

This is a very spicy soup for those who enjoy the flavor of curry.
It is an excellent recipe for a low-fat diet.

PREPARATION TIME: 8 minutes • COOKING TIME: 1 hour
YIELD: 6 servings

1 large onion, peeled and cut into small cubes

1 large carrot, peeled and cut into small cubes

1 stick celery, finely chopped

2 potatoes, peeled and cut into small cubes

$2^2/_3$ cups garden-fresh green peas

1 tablespoon finely chopped mint

8 cups water

1 tablespoon gluten-free curry powder, as desired

1 teaspoon gluten-free concentrated vegetable stock

$^1/_4$ teaspoon each of dried basil, oregano, mixed herbs, nutmeg

1. Place all the ingredients into a large saucepan.

2. Simmer with lid on until vegetables are soft (approximately 1 hour).

3. Blend in an electric food processor or blender or rub through a sieve or food mill.

4. Reheat to serve.

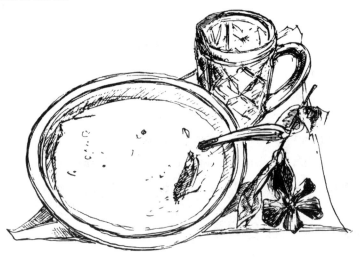

MEATBALL SOUP

This very tasty soup has lots of nutritious ingredients for a hearty winter meal. Serve hot, sprinkled with freshly grated parmesan cheese.

PREPARATION TIME: **20 minutes** • COOKING TIME: **40 minutes**
YIELD: **6–8 servings**

Meatballs

1 lb lean minced steak

1 onion, peeled and finely chopped

1 egg, lightly beaten

$2/3$ cup soft gluten-free bread crumbs or crushed rice cakes

1 tablespoon finely chopped parsley

Freshly ground black pepper, as desired

Maize corn flour (for rolling meatballs)

2 tablespoons salt-reduced monounsaturated margarine

Soup

8 cups water

6 gluten-free beef stock cubes

$3\frac{1}{2}$ oz tomato paste (no added salt)

1 clove garlic, peeled and crushed

2 onions, peeled and roughly chopped

1 carrot, peeled and cut into small cubes

1 medium-sized potato, peeled and cut into small cubes

1 lb can peeled tomatoes (no added salt)

$\frac{1}{4}$ teaspoon freshly ground black pepper

$\frac{1}{2}$ teaspoon dried oregano

$\frac{1}{2}$ teaspoon dried basil

3 bay leaves

$1\frac{1}{3}$ cups gluten-free soy pasta shells

1. To make the meatballs, place minced steak into a medium-sized mixing bowl. Add remaining ingredients except corn flour and margarine and mix well.

2. Shape meat mixture into balls the size of a walnut.

3. Place corn flour into a shallow dish. Roll meatballs in corn flour.

4. Heat margarine in a large saucepan and fry meatballs until golden brown. Drain on absorbent paper.

5. Set meatballs aside while preparing soup.

6. To make the soup, drain any excess margarine from saucepan after cooking meatballs. Place all the ingredients, except meatballs and pasta, into saucepan.

7. Simmer with lid on for 20 minutes.

8. Add meatballs and pasta and simmer for another 20 minutes.

9. Remove bay leaves.

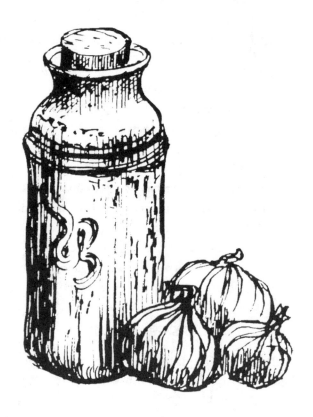

TOMATO SOUP

This is a delicious tomato soup.

PREPARATION TIME: 20 minutes • COOKING TIME: Approximately
30 minutes (approx. 10 minutes in microwave)
YIELD: 4 servings

6 medium-sized ripe tomatoes

$\frac{1}{3}$ cup water

2 large potatoes

1 medium-sized onion

2 tablespoons gluten-free corn flour

1 pint low-fat milk

$\frac{1}{2}$ teaspoon dried basil

$1\frac{1}{2}$ oz tomato paste (no added salt)

1. Place tomatoes into boiling water and leave for 2 minutes. Remove skins. Chop tomatoes roughly and place into a large saucepan with $\frac{1}{3}$ cup water.

2. Peel potatoes and onion and chop roughly. Place into saucepan with tomatoes.

3. Simmer vegetables with lid on until soft.

4. Blend vegetables in an electric food processor or blender or rub through a sieve or food mill.

5. Place corn flour into a small saucepan. Add a little milk and blend well. Gradually stir in remaining milk. Cook over gentle heat, stirring continuously until sauce boils and thickens.

OR Place corn flour into a small microwave-safe bowl. Add a little milk and blend well. Gradually stir in remaining milk. Microwave on high for 1 minute and stir. Continue to microwave on high, stirring at 1 minute intervals until sauce thickens.

6. Pour sauce into blended vegetables and mix well.

7. Stir in basil and tomato paste.

8. Reheat to serve.

BAKED AVOCADO
WITH CRAB

*This recipe is for those who delight in
the flavor of avocado and crab.*

PREPARATION TIME: 20 minutes • COOKING TIME: 5 minutes
YIELD: 6 entrée servings

3 avocados

2 7-oz cans crab flesh

Approximately 2 cups low-fat milk

1 tablespoon salt-reduced
monounsaturated margarine

2 tablespoons maize corn flour

1 teaspoon dill tips

$\frac{1}{4}$ teaspoon each of dried tarragon,
thyme, rosemary, sage

Freshly ground black pepper,
as desired

$\frac{2}{3}$ cup grated low-fat tasty cheese

2 tablespoons freshly grated parmesan cheese

6 small sprigs parsley, for garnish

1. Preheat oven to 400°F.

2. Carefully cut avocados in half lengthwise and remove pits.

3. Place avocado halves into individual ovenproof avocado dishes or place into an ovenproof dish and support with strips of foil.

4. Strain crab flesh and reserve liquid. Pour reserved liquid into a measuring jug. Add sufficient milk to make 2 cups of liquid.

5. Place crab flesh into cavity of avocados.

6. Place margarine into a small saucepan. Melt over a low heat. Remove from heat and stir in corn flour. Return to heat and cook for 1 minute, stirring continuously. Remove from heat. Add a little liquid and blend well. Gradually stir in remaining liquid. Return to heat and cook over a gentle heat, stirring continuously until sauce boils and thickens.

OR Place margarine into a microwave-safe bowl and microwave on high for 30 seconds. Stir in corn flour and microwave on high for 20 seconds. Add a little liquid and blend well. Gradually stir in remaining liquid. Microwave on high for 1 minute and stir. Continue to microwave on high, stirring at 30 second intervals, until sauce thickens.

7. Stir herbs and pepper into sauce.

8. Pour a little sauce over each avocado.

9. Top with grated cheese.

10. Place avocados into oven and cook for approximately 5 minutes, or until cheese has melted and is lightly golden brown. It is important not to cook avocados for too long or flesh will become soft.

11. Garnish with sprigs of parsley and serve immediately.

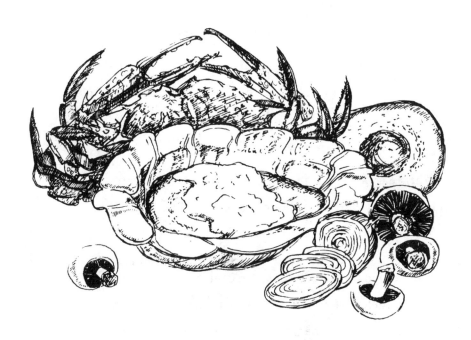

BAKED OMELETTE ROLL

PREPARATION TIME: **15 minutes** • COOKING TIME: **22 minutes**
YIELD: **6 servings with salad**

5 eggs, separated

2 tablespoons cold water

$\frac{1}{2}$ cup gluten-free, plain,
all-purpose flour, sifted

$\frac{1}{4}$ teaspoon dried oregano

2 tablespoons butter or salt-reduced
monounsaturated margarine

2 tablespoons maize corn flour

2 cups milk

$2\frac{2}{3}$ cups grated cheese

$2\frac{2}{3}$ cups diced ham

1 tablespoon finely chopped chives

1. Preheat oven to 350°F.

2. Prepare a 12 x 9-inch flat cake tray by spraying with cooking spray. Line base of tray with baking paper.

3. Place egg whites into a large, dry, clean bowl. Beat until egg whites are stiff.

4. Whisk egg yolks. Stir in cold water. Stir into egg whites.

5. Lightly fold gluten-free flour and oregano into egg.

6. Spread over base of prepared tray.

7. Place into a moderate oven and bake for approximately 15 minutes or until golden brown and set in the center.

8. While omelette is cooking, prepare sauce.

9. Place butter into a medium-sized saucepan. Melt over a low heat.

OR Place butter into a medium-sized microwave-safe bowl. Cover and microwave on high for 1 minute or until butter is melted.

10. Stir corn flour into melted butter.

11. Return saucepan to heat and cook, stirring continuously for 30 seconds.

OR Microwave on high for 30 seconds and stir.

12. Gradually stir in milk.

13. Return to heat and cook until sauce thickens, stirring continuously.

OR Microwave on high for 30 seconds and stir. Continue to microwave on high, stirring at 30 second intervals until sauce thickens.

14. Stir in $\frac{2}{3}$ cup grated cheese, ham, and chives.

15. When omelette is cooked remove from oven and allow to stand for 3 minutes.

16. Spread sauce over omelette. Roll up from wide side. Allow to remain wrapped in baking paper for 5 minutes.

17. Remove baking paper and place omelette roll onto a clean sheet of baking paper on tray.

18. Sprinkle remaining cheese over roll and bake for another 7 minutes until cheese is melted.

19. Slice and serve hot or cold as desired.

PRAWN ASPIC MOLDS

This recipe is excellent for entertaining. The molds are delicious to serve as an appetizer or entrée. Larger molds can be used if desired.

PREPARATION TIME: 20 minutes
(allow time for molds to set, about 2 hours)
YIELD: 15 small molds

2 tablespoons finely diced carrot

2 tablespoons finely diced pumpkin

2 tablespoons finely chopped snow peas

2 tablespoons finely chopped celery

7 oz can peeled prawns

1 lb can asparagus cuts

2 tablespoons cold water

2 x $\frac{1}{3}$ oz packets gelatin

1 teaspoon concentrated
gluten-free vegetable stock

Freshly ground black pepper, as desired

Lettuce leaves, for serving

1. Lightly steam carrot, pumpkin, snow peas, and celery.

OR Place carrot, pumpkin, snow peas, and celery onto a flat microwave-safe plate. Cover with vented plastic wrap and microwave on high for 1 minute.

2. Strain liquid from prawns and asparagus, and reserve liquids.

3. Pour cold water into a small bowl. Stir in gelatin and leave for 2 minutes.

4. Pour reserved liquids from prawns and asparagus into a measuring jug. Make up to $2\frac{2}{3}$ cups of liquid with boiling water. Add vegetable stock and stir until dissolved. Stir in freshly ground black pepper. Pour into soaked gelatin.

5. Place soaked gelatin into a small saucepan. Cook over a gentle heat until liquid boils and gelatin dissolves. Allow to cool slightly.

OR Place soaked gelatin into a small microwave-safe bowl and microwave for approximately 1 minute on high or until liquid boils and gelatin dissolves. Allow to cool slightly.

6. Place 15 small molds onto a flat tray to facilitate handling.

7. Arrange prawns attractively in bottom of molds. Pour a small quantity of liquid over prawns. Place molds into refrigerator and allow to set (approximately 5–10 minutes).

8. Remove molds from refrigerator and arrange vegetables in molds. Pour remaining liquid evenly into molds.

9. Refrigerate molds until firm (at least 2 hours or overnight).

10. To serve, dip each mold in hot water for a couple of seconds and unmold onto a bed of lettuce.

SARDINE DIP

This dip is very easy to make and is suitable to serve, with rice crackers, at a party. It needs to be made at least 2 hours before it is required. It is best made the night before to allow full development of flavor.

PREPARATION TIME: 5 minutes (+ 2 or more hours)

8 oz package light cream cheese
$3\frac{1}{3}$ oz can gluten-free sardines
Finely grated rind and juice of $\frac{1}{2}$ a lemon
1 clove garlic, peeled and crushed
1 tablespoon finely chopped parsley
$\frac{1}{4}$ teaspoon freshly ground black pepper

1. Place all ingredients into the bowl of an electric food processor or blender and mix until smooth (or beat ingredients well by hand).

2. Pour into a serving bowl.

3. Seal bowl and refrigerate overnight (or at least 2 hours) before serving.

Salmon Pâté

This is a very tasty pâté served with rice crackers. It can be served with pre-dinner drinks or as an entrée. It is necessary to make this pâté the day before it is required. Freshly cooked salmon can be used in place of canned salmon.

PREPARATION TIME: 20 minutes

YIELD: 6–8 entrée servings

1 lb can pink salmon

3 tablespoons cold water

$\frac{1}{3}$ oz packet gelatin

$\frac{2}{3}$ cup chopped shallots

$\frac{2}{3}$ cup dry white wine

1 teaspoon gluten-free
concentrated vegetable stock

8 oz package light cream cheese

Freshly ground black pepper, as desired

1 tablespoon chopped mint

Lettuce leaves, for serving

1. Lightly oil a medium-sized mold or basin suitable for pâté.

2. Remove bones from salmon and discard. Place salmon and liquid into the bowl of an electric food processor or blender.

3. Place water into a small saucepan and stir in gelatin. Allow to stand for 2 minutes. Heat over a low heat to melt gelatin. Pour into blender.

OR Place water into a small microwave-safe bowl and stir in gelatin. Allow to stand for 2 minutes. Microwave on high for 1 minute. Pour into blender.

4. Add remaining ingredients and blend until smooth.

5. Pour into prepared mold.

6. Cover and refrigerate overnight.

7. To serve, unmold onto a bed of lettuce leaves.

SMOKED SALMON SUSHI

Sushi is usually made with raw fish; however, this recipe uses smoked salmon. It is a nice variation to the traditional recipe.

PREPARATION TIME: 40 minutes (includes 10 minutes cooling time)
COOKING TIME: 15 minutes

YIELD: 6 servings

$2\frac{2}{3}$ cups basmati rice

4 cups cold water

$\frac{2}{3}$ cup rice wine

2 tablespoons sugar

Pinch of salt, as desired

6 nori sheets

$1\frac{1}{2}$ tablespoons gluten-free light mayonnaise

$\frac{1}{2}$ teaspoon wasabi paste

1 avocado

2 tablespoons lemon juice

$7\frac{1}{2}$ oz smoked salmon

$\frac{2}{3}$ cup gluten-free soy sauce

2 tablespoons mirin

1. Wash rice and drain.

2. Combine rice and water in a saucepan. Cover with a lid and bring to a boil. Reduce heat and cook with lid on for 12 minutes or until all the water is absorbed and rice is tender. Remove from heat. Leave lid on and allow to cool slightly. Rice must be thoroughly cooked so sushi will hold together.

OR Place rice and water into a microwave rice steamer. Microwave on high for 2 minutes. Continue to microwave on medium-high for about 5 minutes or until rice is tender.

3. Combine rice wine, sugar, and salt in a medium-sized bowl. Gradually add to cooked rice and stir well. If rice mixture appears a little too wet, do not add any more liquid. Rice must be allowed to cool completely before rolling up for sushi.

4. Place a sushi mat on a clean work bench. Slats must run horizontally.

5. Place a nori sheet, shiny side down on the mat. Make sure the sheet is 1 inch from the side of the mat closest to you.

6. Using wet hands, spread 1 cup rice over the nori sheet, leaving a $1\frac{1}{4}$-inch border along the edge farthest from you.

7. Place mayonnaise and wasabi into a small bowl. Mix well to combine ingredients.

8. Peel avocado. Cut into thin slices and brush with lemon juice.

9. Spread a little wasabi mixture along the center of the rice. Add slices of avocado and salmon.

10. Pick up the edge of the mat closest to you. Hold filling in place while rolling the mat over to enclose the rice and filling in the nori sheet.

11. Repeat with the remaining nori sheets, rice, and filling to make five more rolls.

12. Combine the soy sauce and mirin in a small jug.

13. Cut sushi rolls into 1-inch rolls and place onto a platter for serving.

14. Just before serving pour mirin sauce over rolls.

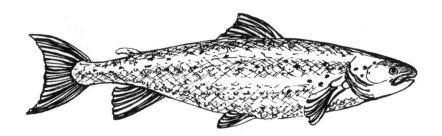

6.

Main Courses

Meat

Chinese Beef, 56

Easy Quiche, 57

Greek-Style Lasagna, 58

Ham Pie, 60

Hawaiian Pizza, 62

Meatballs with Yogurt Dipping Sauce, 64

Moussaka, 65

Pork Chops with Carrot and Orange Sauce, 66

Rib Steak with Mustard Sauce, 67

Shepherd's Pie, 68

Steak with Apple and Wine Sauce, 70

Sweet Curry, 71

Tacos, 72

Taco Sauce, 73

Veal Casserole, 74

Veal Pie, 75

Chicken

Chicken in Red and White Wine, 77

Chicken and Broccoli, 79

Chicken Casserole, 80

Chicken with Cherry Sauce, 81

Chicken and Pineapple, 83

Coconut Lime Chicken, 84

Cranberry Citrus Chicken, 86

Seafood

Salmon Pie, 87

Tuna Casserole, 89

Tuna Mornay, 91

MEAT

CHINESE BEEF

This recipe is a delicious way of preparing beef, Chinese style. The vegetables are cooked just long enough to keep them crisp. Serve with rice or salad.

PREPARATION TIME: **20 minutes** • COOKING TIME: **Approximately 10 minutes**
YIELD: **6 servings**

2 lbs best-quality lean rump steak

3 tablespoons red wine

$\frac{1}{2}$ teaspoon baking soda

1 tablespoon gluten-free soy sauce

1 teaspoon ground ginger

1 teaspoon gluten-free mild prepared mustard

1 teaspoon gluten-free curry powder

1 tablespoon raw sugar

1 tablespoon olive oil

1 carrot

1 zucchini

1 stick celery

1 red bell pepper

1 onion

2 tablespoons maize corn flour

2 cups gluten-free beef stock

1 tablespoon gluten-free soy sauce, extra

1. Cut rump steak into thin strips.

2. Place meat into a large bowl. Stir in red wine, baking soda, soy sauce, ginger, mustard, curry, and sugar. Cover bowl and marinate in refrigerator overnight.

3. The next day, drain meat and discard liquid.

4. Heat oil in a wok or frying pan.

5. Add portion of meat to wok and cook until just tender. Set meat aside and keep warm.

6. Repeat step 5 until all meat is cooked.

7. Prepare vegetables as necessary and cut into thin strips.

8. Add vegetables to wok and toss until lightly cooked.

9. Place corn flour into a small bowl. Add a little beef stock and blend well. Gradually stir in remaining beef stock and extra soy sauce.

10. Pour sauce into wok with vegetables. Stir for 1 minute to cook sauce.

11. Add meat and heat through.

EASY QUICHE

This recipe will suit the cook who wants a good-quality finished product with a minimum of effort. Serve with salad.

PREPARATION TIME: 8 minutes • COOKING TIME: 30 minutes
(12 minutes in microwave)
YIELD: 4–6 servings

1 lb can salmon (drain and discard liquid)
1 large onion, peeled and finely chopped
2 teaspoons finely chopped parsley
$1\frac{2}{3}$ cups gluten-free bread crumbs
$1\frac{1}{3}$ cups grated low-fat tasty cheese
Freshly ground black pepper, as desired
$1\frac{1}{3}$ cups low-fat warm milk
$\frac{2}{3}$ cup light sour cream
3 eggs, lightly beaten
1 teaspoon gluten-free mustard

1. Preheat oven to 350°F.

2. Prepare a quiche dish by spraying with cooking spray.

3. Spread salmon over base of prepared dish.

4. Place remaining ingredients into a medium-sized mixing bowl and mix to combine. Pour over salmon.

5. Bake for approximately 30 minutes or until cooked when tested.

OR Microwave on medium-high for approximately 12 minutes or until cooked when tested. Allow to stand for 5 minutes before serving.

GREEK-STYLE LASAGNA

This tasty lasagna can be prepared the day before it is required and baked on the day for serving.

PREPARATION TIME: 20 minutes • COOKING TIME: 40 minutes

YIELD: 6 servings

Base

2 tomatoes

2 tablespoons olive oil

1 large onion, peeled and finely chopped

1 clove garlic, peeled and crushed

8 mushrooms, cut into thin slices

$\frac{1}{2}$ teaspoon dried oregano

$\frac{1}{2}$ teaspoon dried basil

6 small eggplants, cut into $\frac{1}{2}$-inch slices

1 tablespoon olive oil, extra

1 lb minced lamb (or beef)

7 oz box Orgran Rice and Corn Lasagna Mini Sheets (gluten-free)

Sauce

8 oz package light cream cheese

$1\frac{1}{3}$ cups low-fat natural yogurt

3 eggs, lightly beaten

4 oz grated reduced-fat cheddar cheese

2 tablespoons finely grated parmesan cheese

1. Preheat oven to 400°F.

2. Prepare a large, flat baking dish by spraying with cooking spray.

3. Place tomatoes into a small bowl. Cover with boiling water. Leave for 2–3 minutes. Remove skins and cut tomatoes into $\frac{1}{2}$-inch cubes.

4. Pour oil into a medium-sized frying pan. Heat over a gentle heat. Add tomatoes, onions, garlic, and mushrooms. Add herbs and sauté for about 3–5 minutes. Add sliced eggplant.

5. In a separate pan add extra oil. Heat over a gentle heat. Add meat and cook until meat is brown.

6. Prepare lasagna sheets according to directions on package.

7. Line the base of the dish with lasagna sheets. Spread half the meat over the lasagna sheets. Place another layer of lasagna sheets on meat. Spread remaining meat over lasagna sheets. Top with cooked vegetables. Top with any remaining lasagna sheets.

8. To make the sauce, place cream cheese into a small bowl. Beat until soft and smooth. Stir in yogurt and eggs.

9. Spread sauce over ingredients in baking dish. Sprinkle with grated cheeses.

10. Place the dish into a moderately hot oven and bake for approximately 40 minutes or until heated through.

11. When cooked, remove from oven and serve hot or cold as desired.

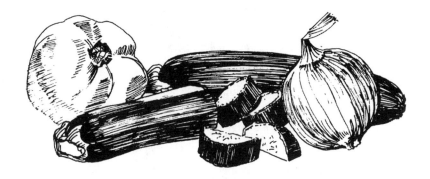

HAM PIE

This is a delicious ham pie. It can be made if you have leftover ham.
Serve hot or cold with salad.

PREPARATION TIME: **20 minutes** • COOKING TIME: **45 minutes**
YIELD: **6–8 servings**

Pastry

²/₃ cup buckwheat flour

²/₃ cup white rice flour

²/₃ cup gluten-free, plain, all-purpose flour

¹/₃ cup soy flour

2 teaspoons gluten-free baking powder

²/₃ cup ground rice

3 tablespoons salt-reduced
monounsaturated margarine

Water to moisten dry ingredients
(approximately ¹/₃ cup)

Filling

2 medium-sized potatoes

1 lb lean ham cut from the bone

1 medium-sized onion,
peeled and finely diced

3 eggs, lightly beaten

1¹/₃ cups low-fat milk

2 packets gluten-free soup mix,
vegetable flavor

8 oz package light cream cheese

1¹/₃ cups grated low-fat tasty cheese

2 tablespoons freshly grated parmesan cheese

2 tablespoons finely chopped parsley

8 cherry tomatoes

Pastry

1. Preheat oven to 400°F.

2. Prepare a 9-inch pie dish by spraying with cooking spray.

3. Sift flours and baking powder into a medium-sized mixing bowl. Stir in ground rice.

4. Rub margarine into dry ingredients until mixture resembles fine bread crumbs. This process may be done by hand or with the aid of an electric food processor.

5. Stir in sufficient water to mix to a firm dough.

6. Turn dough out onto a lightly floured (gluten-free) board and knead lightly.

7. Gently roll pastry to approximately $\frac{1}{4}$-inch thickness to fit base and sides of dish.

8. Carefully line base and sides of prepared pie dish with pastry.

Filling

1. Peel and dice potatoes.

2. Place potato into a steamer and cook until potato is just tender. Do not overcook or potato will break up. Set potato aside.

OR Spread potato over a large, flat microwave-safe plate. Cover with vented plastic wrap. Microwave on high for approximately 3 minutes or until potato is tender.

3. Cut ham into small cubes and place into pie plate.

4. Place onion on ham.

5. Place cooked potato into pie plate with ham and onion.

6. Pour egg into a medium-sized mixing bowl. Add milk, soup mix, cheeses, and parsley and stir well.

7. Pour filling into pie plate. Decorate top of pie with any remaining pastry. Place tomatoes evenly around pie.

8. Place pie into oven and cook for approximately 45 minutes or until set in the center when tested.

HAWAIIAN PIZZA

A recipe for a pizza is a popular inclusion in a recipe book.
This pizza base is made with gluten-free products.
Serve with salad.

PREPARATION TIME: 20 minutes • COOKING TIME: 20 minutes
YIELD: 6 servings

Base

$2/3$ cup Orgran gluten-free pizza mix

$2/3$ cup white rice flour

2 teaspoons gluten-free baking powder

2 tablespoons salt-reduced
monounsaturated margarine

$1/3$ cup water

1 egg yolk

Topping

$3\frac{1}{2}$ oz tomato paste

$1\frac{1}{3}$ cups chopped light leg ham

$1\frac{1}{3}$ cups pineapple pieces
in natural juice, drained

1 stick celery, finely chopped

2 tomatoes, cut into small cubes

$1/3$ cup chopped olives

$2/3$ cup chopped shallots

$1\frac{1}{3}$ cups grated low-fat tasty cheese

1 tablespoon freshly grated
parmesan cheese

1. Preheat oven to 400°F.

2. Prepare a 12-inch pizza tray by spraying with cooking spray.

3. Sift pizza mix, flour, and baking powder into a medium-sized mixing
   bowl.

4. Rub margarine into sifted dry ingredients until mixture resembles fine bread crumbs. This process may be done by hand or with the aid of an electric food processor.

5. Whisk water and egg yolk in a small bowl. Pour liquid into dry ingredients and mix to a firm dough.

6. Turn dough out onto a lightly floured (gluten-free) board and knead lightly. Roll out to approximately $1/4$-inch thickness to fit base of tray.

7. Cut into 2-inch-wide strips. Place strips of pastry onto prepared pizza tray and press into position.

8. Place topping ingredients onto pastry base in order listed above.

9. Place pizza into oven and bake for approximately 20 minutes or until golden brown and pastry is cooked.

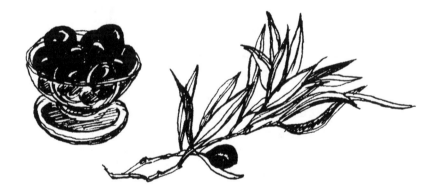

MEATBALLS WITH YOGURT DIPPING SAUCE

PREPARATION TIME: 20 minutes • COOKING TIME: 15 minutes
YIELD: Approximately 24 small meatballs

Meatballs

1 lb lean minced beef

$1\frac{1}{3}$ cups fine gluten-free bread crumbs

1 egg, lightly beaten

1 medium red onion, peeled and finely chopped

$\frac{1}{3}$ cup finely chopped pine nuts

2 tablespoons finely chopped fresh parsley

2 tablespoons finely chopped fresh mint

1 tablespoon finely chopped fresh coriander

1 clove garlic, peeled and crushed

$\frac{1}{2}$ teaspoon ground cumin

$\frac{1}{4}$ teaspoon ground nutmeg

Gluten-free, plain, all-purpose flour, to toss meatballs

Olive oil, for deep frying

Yogurt Dipping Sauce

$\frac{1}{2}$ teaspoon finely chopped red chili, as desired

2 tablespoons finely chopped fresh parsley

2 tablespoons finely chopped fresh mint

1 tablespoon finely chopped fresh coriander

1 clove garlic, peeled and crushed

16 oz light natural yogurt

1. To make the meatballs, mix all the ingredients, except flour and oil, well together. Shape small portions approximately the size of a walnut. Toss each meatball in gluten-free plain flour. Heat a quantity of oil in a deep-frying pan. Fry a portion of meatballs until golden brown. Drain on absorbent paper. Fry remaining meatballs and drain.

2. To make the yogurt dipping sauce, place all the ingredients into the bowl of an electric blender and blend until smooth.

3. Serve meatballs hot or cold with yogurt dipping sauce.

MOUSSAKA

Eggplant is the traditional vegetable used for moussaka.
This recipe uses small finger-shaped slices of eggplant.

PREPARATION TIME: 20 minutes • COOKING TIME: 40 minutes
YIELD: 6 servings

2 tomatoes
2 tablespoons olive oil
1 large onion, peeled and finely chopped
1 clove garlic, peeled and crushed
8 mushrooms, cut into thin slices
$\frac{1}{2}$ teaspoon dried oregano
$\frac{1}{2}$ teaspoon dried basil
6 small eggplants, cut into $\frac{1}{2}$-inch slices
1 tablespoon olive oil, extra
1 lb minced lamb (or beef)
$1\frac{1}{3}$ cups cooked basmati rice
4 oz grated low-fat cheddar cheese

Sauce
4 oz light cream cheese
$1\frac{1}{3}$ cups low-fat natural yogurt
2 eggs, lightly beaten
1 tablespoon finely chopped parsley
4 oz grated low-fat cheddar cheese
2 tablespoons finely grated parmesan cheese

1. Preheat oven to 400°F.

2. Prepare a large, flat baking dish by spraying with cooking spray.

3. Place tomatoes into a small bowl. Cover with boiling water. Leave for 2–3 minutes. Remove skins and cut tomatoes into $\frac{1}{2}$-inch cubes.

4. Pour oil into a medium-sized frying pan. Heat over a gentle heat. Add tomato, onion, garlic, and mushrooms. Add herbs and sauté for about 3–5 minutes. Add sliced eggplant.

5. In a separate pan add extra oil. Heat over a gentle heat. Add meat and cook until meat is brown.

6. Place a layer of meat into prepared dish. Top with half the cooked vegetables, half the rice, and half the grated cheese.

7. Repeat with a layer of meat, vegetable, rice, and cheese.

8. To make the sauce, place cream cheese into a small bowl. Beat until soft and smooth. Stir in yogurt, egg, and parsley. Spread over ingredients in baking dish. Sprinkle with grated cheeses.

9. Place dish into a moderate oven and bake for approximately 40 minutes or until heated through.

10. When cooked, remove from oven and serve hot or allow to cool and serve cold.

PORK CHOPS WITH CARROT AND ORANGE SAUCE

The delicious flavor of pork is enhanced with the addition of a tasty sauce. Serve on a bed of cooked rice.

PREPARATION TIME: 5 minutes
COOKING TIME: Approximately 15 minutes
YIELD: 6 servings

6 butterfly pork chops (all fat removed)
4 small carrots, diced
Juice of 1 orange combined with water
to make $1\frac{1}{3}$ cups liquid
1 tablespoon finely chopped raw ginger

1. Cook pork chops in a nonstick frying pan until lightly golden brown and tender.

2. While chops are cooking, place carrots and liquid into a small saucepan. Cook over a gentle heat with lid on until carrots are tender; add ginger and stir well. Blend in an electric food processor or blender, or rub through a sieve or food mill.

3. Serve sauce over cooked chops.

RIB STEAK WITH MUSTARD SAUCE

Best-quality rib-eye fillet steaks are used in this recipe.
If you wish you can use rump steak as a substitute.
Serve with rice, vegetables, or salad.

PREPARATION TIME: 15 minutes (steak is best marinated overnight)
COOKING TIME: Approximately 10 minutes
YIELD: 4 servings

4 thick rib-eye fillet steaks (all fat removed)
$2^2/_3$ cups gluten-free beef stock
2 teaspoons prepared hot mustard
(gluten-free)
$1/_3$ cup white wine
Freshly ground black pepper, as desired
2 teaspoons olive oil
3 tablespoons maize corn flour
$1^1/_3$ cups gluten-free soy drink

1. Place steaks into a shallow container.

2. In a small bowl, combine stock, mustard, wine, and pepper and pour over steaks. Cover and marinate in refrigerator overnight, turning steaks once if possible.

3. The next day, drain steaks and reserve marinade.

4. Pour oil into a nonstick frying pan. Heat pan over a high heat. Add steaks and sear on both sides. Reduce heat and cook until steaks are tender, turning frequently.

5. Remove steaks from pan. Set aside and keep warm.

6. Place corn flour into a small bowl. Blend with a little reserved marinade. Add remaining marinade and soy drink.

7. Pour liquid into pan. Cook over a gentle heat, stirring continuously until sauce thickens.

8. Pour sauce over steak for serving.

SHEPHERD'S PIE

This is a traditional recipe that has been around for many years.
A friend of mine, Aili, asked me to give her a recipe for
a gluten-free shepherd's pie. I trust Aili along
with many others will enjoy this recipe.

PREPARATION TIME: 20 minutes • COOKING TIME: 40 minutes
(8 minutes in microwave)

YIELD: 6 servings

6 large potatoes

2 tablespoons skim milk, approximately
(for mashing potato)

1 tablespoon butter or monounsaturated
salt-reduced margarine
(for mashing potato)

Salt, as desired (for mashing potato)

Freshly ground black pepper, as desired
(for mashing potato)

1 lb finely minced baked lamb

1 onion, peeled and finely chopped

$\frac{1}{2}$ teaspoon dried mixed herbs

1 tablespoon finely chopped parsley

Salt, extra, as desired

$\frac{1}{2}$ teaspoon freshly ground black pepper

$\frac{1}{4}$ teaspoon ground nutmeg

2 tablespoons gluten-free tomato relish
or tomato sauce

1 rasher bacon

$\frac{2}{3}$ cup grated low-fat cheddar cheese

1 egg

1. Preheat oven to 400°F.

2. Prepare a 10-inch pie dish by spraying with cooking spray.

3. Peel potatoes and cut into small cubes. Place into boiling salted water and cook until potatoes are soft.

OR Place potato cubes into the top of a steamer and steam until potatoes are soft.

4. Drain and mash with a little milk, butter, salt, and pepper as desired. Line bottom of pie dish with half the mashed potato.

5. Combine meat, onion, herbs, salt (as desired), pepper, nutmeg, and tomato relish and mix well.

6. Place seasoned meat onto potato in pie dish.

7. Place the remainder of the mashed potato on top of the meat.

8. Remove fat and rind from bacon and discard. Cut meat into long thin strips. Decorate top of pie with bacon strips.

9. Sprinkle pie with grated cheese.

10. Beat egg and pour over the cheese.

11. Place into a moderately hot oven and bake for approximately 40 minutes or until heated through and golden brown on top.

OR Microwave on high for approximately 8 minutes or until heated through.

12. When cooked, remove from oven. Serve hot or cold as desired with vegetables or salad.

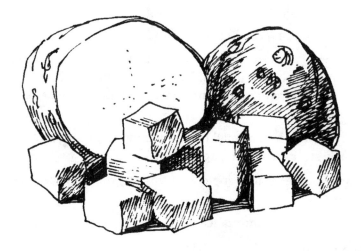

STEAK WITH APPLE AND WINE SAUCE

This recipe uses prime-quality beef and is low in added fat.
Serve garnished with freshly ground black pepper and
accompanied by vegetables and/or salad.

PREPARATION TIME: **8 minutes**
COOKING TIME: **Approximately 10 minutes**
YIELD: **4 servings**

4 thick top-quality fillet steaks
(all fat removed)

1⅓ cups apple juice (no added sugar)

⅓ cup white wine

1 teaspoon olive oil

1 tablespoon maize corn flour

1⅓ cups apple juice, extra

1 teaspoon finely chopped fresh ginger

¼ teaspoon dried sage

1 green cooking apple, peeled and grated

Freshly ground black pepper, as desired

⅓ cup white wine, extra

1. Place steaks into a large bowl. Pour in apple juice and wine. Cover and marinate in refrigerator overnight.

2. The next day, drain steaks and discard liquid.

3. Pour oil into a nonstick frying pan. Heat pan over a high heat. Add steaks and sear on both sides. Reduce heat and cook until steaks are tender, turning frequently. Remove steaks from pan. Set aside and keep warm.

4. Place corn flour into a small bowl. Blend with a little extra apple juice. Gradually stir in remaining apple juice.

5. Stir ginger, sage, grated apple, and freshly ground black pepper. Pour into pan.

6. Stir over a low heat until sauce thickens. Stir in extra wine.

7. Serve sauce over steak.

Sweet Curry

This curry has a delicious fruity flavor. You can make it hotter to your liking by adding a stronger mustard and more curry if you wish. Serve on a bed of rice sprinkled with chopped parsley and wedges of lemon.

PREPARATION TIME: 15 minutes • COOKING TIME: 40 minutes
(50 minutes in microwave)
YIELD: 6 servings

2 lbs lean veal
2 tablespoons maize corn flour
$\frac{1}{2}$ cup chopped dried apricots
$\frac{1}{2}$ cup golden raisins (sultanas)
$\frac{1}{2}$ cup chopped raisins
$\frac{1}{3}$ cup chopped shallots
2 teaspoons gluten-free prepared mild mustard
1 teaspoon gluten-free curry powder
$\frac{2}{3}$ cup sweet white wine
2 teaspoons gluten-free Worcestershire sauce
1 tablespoon gluten-free soy sauce
1 tablespoon honey

1. Prepare a medium-sized casserole dish by spraying with cooking spray.

2. Cut veal into small cubes.

3. Place corn flour into a small bowl. Lightly toss veal cubes in corn flour and place into prepared casserole dish.

4. Place apricots, raisins, and shallots over veal cubes in casserole dish.

5. Mix mustard, curry, wine, sauces, and honey in a small bowl. Pour into casserole dish.

6. Cover and marinate in refrigerator overnight.

7. The next day, place curry into a cold oven. Turn oven to 350°F and cook for approximately 40 minutes or until veal cubes are tender.

OR The next day, place curry into a microwave oven. Microwave on low for approximately 50 minutes or until veal cubes are tender. (Although it takes longer to cook the casserole when using the microwave oven, there are the advantages of using less power and the clean up being easier.)

TACOS

*Tacos are very popular for a quick meal. They are suitable
for a gluten-free diet if the shells are made from corn.
Always check ingredients to be sure. Taco sauce can be made
ahead of time to serve with the tacos (see following recipe).*

PREPARATION TIME: 15 minutes
COOKING TIME: Approximately 8 minutes
YIELD: 6 servings

1 large onion

1 teaspoon olive oil

1 lb lean minced steak

1 tablespoon tomato paste (no added salt)

1 tablespoon gluten-free soy sauce

1 tablespoon gluten-free black bean sauce

$\frac{1}{2}$ teaspoon crushed garlic

$\frac{1}{2}$ teaspoon dried oregano

$\frac{1}{4}$ teaspoon dried sage

6 gluten-free taco shells

$2\frac{2}{3}$ cups shredded lettuce

2 tomatoes, cut into $\frac{1}{2}$-inch cubes

18 slices cucumber

2 cups grated low-fat cheese

1. Peel and finely chop onion.

2. Pour oil onto a nonstick frying pan. Add onion and cook over a medium heat until lightly golden brown.

3. Add minced steak, tomato paste, soy sauce, black bean sauce, garlic, oregano, and sage. Cook, stirring occasionally, until meat is tender.

4. Spoon seasoned meat into taco shells.

5. Arrange filled taco shells on serving plates with shredded lettuce, tomato cubes, and cucumber slices.

6. Sprinkle grated cheese over taco shells.

TACO SAUCE

My daughter Maria made up this recipe and it has
been a family favorite. Serve with tacos.

PREPARATION TIME: 15 minutes • COOKING TIME: 20 minutes
YIELD: Approximately 1 pint

2 large tomatoes

1 clove garlic, peeled and crushed

1 onion, peeled and diced

$\frac{1}{2}$ teaspoon hot paprika

2 tablespoons tomato paste
(no added salt)

3 tablespoons concentrated apple juice
(no added sugar)

3 tablespoons herb or white vinegar

$\frac{1}{2}$ teaspoon Tabasco sauce

1 tablespoon arrowroot or
gluten-free corn flour

1. Place tomatoes into boiling water and leave for 2 minutes. Remove skins.

2. Blend all the ingredients in the bowl of an electric food processor or blender.

3. Place mixture into a small saucepan. Stir over a gentle heat until sauce boils. Simmer until sauce reduces and thickens.

OR Place mixture into a small microwave-safe bowl. Microwave on high for 2 minutes and stir. Continue to microwave on high, stirring at 2 minute intervals, until sauce boils and thickens.

4. When cooked, bottle while still hot and seal. Sauce will keep for up to one week in the refrigerator.

VEAL CASSEROLE

Tender cubes of veal, together with vegetables, make this a nutritious casserole. Serve with cooked rice and salad.

PREPARATION TIME: 15 minutes • COOKING TIME: $1\frac{1}{2}$ hours
(1 hour in microwave)
YIELD: 6 servings

1 lb lean veal fillets,
cut into small cubes

1 carrot, peeled and diced

1 potato, peeled and diced

1 can gluten-free tomato soup

1 stick celery, finely chopped

1 tablespoon finely chopped
red bell pepper

1 onion, peeled and finely chopped

$\frac{1}{3}$ cup white wine

2 tablespoons ground rice

$\frac{1}{2}$ teaspoon dried mixed herbs

1. Preheat oven to 325°F.

2. Prepare a 4-pint casserole dish by spraying with cooking spray.

3. Mix all the ingredients in a medium-sized bowl. Place into prepared casserole dish.

4. Place casserole into oven and cook for approximately $1\frac{1}{2}$ hours or until meat and vegetables are tender.

OR Microwave on medium-low for approximately 1 hour or until meat and vegetables are tender. Stir occasionally during cooking.

VEAL PIE

A lot of people enjoy a meat pie. This pie uses lean veal.
Serve hot with vegetables.

PREPARATION TIME: 25 minutes • COOKING TIME: 30 minutes
YIELD: 6 servings

Filling

1 lb lean minced veal

1 onion, peeled and finely grated

$3\frac{1}{2}$ oz tomato paste (no added salt)

$\frac{1}{2}$ cup tomato sauce

2 tablespoons gluten-free
Worcestershire sauce

$\frac{1}{2}$ teaspoon dried basil

$\frac{1}{4}$ teaspoon each of nutmeg,
dried sage, dried rosemary

Pastry

$\frac{2}{3}$ cup buckwheat flour

$\frac{2}{3}$ cup white rice flour

$\frac{2}{3}$ cup gluten-free, plain, all-purpose flour

2 teaspoons gluten-free baking powder

6 tablespoons salt-reduced
monounsaturated margarine

$\frac{1}{2}$ cup water

1 egg yolk

1 teaspoon lemon juice

$\frac{2}{3}$ cup grated low-fat cheese

1. Preheat oven to 400°F. Prepare a 9-inch pie plate by spraying with cooking spray.

2. To make the filling, place all the filling ingredients into a medium-sized saucepan and cook with lid on over a gentle heat for 5 minutes, stirring occasionally. Allow to cool slightly.

3. Sift flours and baking powder into a medium-sized mixing bowl.

4. Rub margarine into sifted dry ingredients until mixture resembles fine bread crumbs. This process may be done by hand or with the aid of an electric food processor.

5. Whisk water, egg yolk, and lemon juice in a small bowl. Pour liquid into dry ingredients and mix to a firm dough.

6. Turn dough out onto a lightly floured (gluten-free) board and knead lightly. Divide pastry into thirds. Carefully roll two-thirds of the pastry to approximately $\frac{1}{4}$-inch thickness to fit base and sides of pie plate.

7. Carefully line base and sides of prepared pie plate with rolled-out pastry.

8. Place veal filling into prepared pastry case.

9. Carefully roll out remainder of pastry and place over filling.

10. Sprinkle grated cheese on top of pastry.

11. Place pie into oven and cook for 10 minutes. Reduce heat to 325°F and cook for another 20 minutes or until golden brown and pastry is cooked.

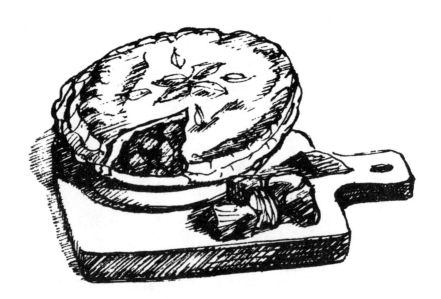

CHICKEN

CHICKEN IN RED AND WHITE WINE

This is a superb recipe to serve at a dinner party. The best flavor results will be produced by marinating overnight. However, it is possible to prepare and cook this recipe immediately. Serve with rice, vegetables, or salad.

PREPARATION TIME: 20 minutes (+ marinate overnight)
COOKING TIME: 2 hours
YIELD: 6 servings

2 lbs chicken fillets
(skin and fat removed)

$\frac{1}{3}$ cup red wine

$\frac{1}{3}$ cup white wine

$1\frac{1}{3}$ cups gluten-free chicken stock

Finely grated rind and juice of $\frac{1}{2}$ a lemon

Maize corn flour for rolling
(approx. $1\frac{1}{3}$ cups)

Olive oil for frying (approx. $\frac{1}{3}$ cup)

2 tablespoons maize corn flour

$1\frac{1}{3}$ cups apricot nectar (no added sugar)

$1\frac{1}{3}$ cups gluten-free chicken stock, extra

1. Cut chicken fillets into small cubes. Place chicken cubes into a large bowl.

2. Pour wine and stock over chicken cubes. Add rind and juice of lemon to chicken cubes. Cover and marinate in refrigerator overnight.

3. The next day, strain chicken cubes and discard juices. Remove excess moisture from chicken cubes on absorbent kitchen paper.

4. Place corn flour into a small bowl. Lightly toss chicken cubes in corn flour.

5. Heat a little olive oil in a nonstick frying pan. Place a few chicken cubes into pan. Cook, turning frequently, until chicken cubes are golden brown and cooked. Place cooked chicken cubes into an ovenproof serving dish. Continue to follow these steps until all the chicken cubes are cooked, using more oil if needed.

6. Place the corn flour into a small saucepan. Add a little apricot nectar and blend well. Gradually stir in remaining apricot nectar and chicken stock. Cook over a low heat, stirring continuously until sauce boils and thickens.

OR Place the corn flour into a small microwave-safe bowl. Add a little apricot nectar and blend well. Gradually stir in remaining apricot nectar and chicken stock. Microwave on high for 30 seconds and stir. Continue to microwave on high, stirring at 30 second intervals until sauce thickens.

7. Pour sauce over cooked chicken cubes.

8. Reheat in oven at 400°F for 5 minutes before serving.

OR Reheat on medium-high for 2 minutes before serving.

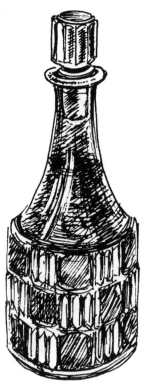

CHICKEN AND BROCCOLI

*This recipe has a delicious combination of chicken, broccoli, and celery.
Serve with rice and/or salad.*

PREPARATION TIME: 12 minutes • COOKING TIME: 30 minutes
(20 minutes in microwave)
YIELD: 4–6 servings

6 chicken fillets (skin and fat removed)

2 tablespoons maize corn flour

2 packets gluten-free soup mix,
vegetable flavor

$2\frac{2}{3}$ cups warm water

$\frac{1}{3}$ cup white wine

$\frac{1}{3}$ teaspoon paprika

$1\frac{1}{3}$ cups finely chopped broccoli

$1\frac{1}{3}$ cups finely chopped celery

1 tablespoon finely chopped parsley

1. Prepare a medium-sized casserole dish (with lid) by spraying with cooking spray.

2. Cut chicken fillets into small cubes.

3. Place corn flour into a small bowl. Lightly toss chicken cubes in corn flour and place into prepared casserole dish.

4. Stir in remaining ingredients.

5. Cover and marinate in refrigerator overnight.

6. The next day, place casserole dish (with lid on) into a cold oven. Turn oven to 350°F and cook for approximately 30 minutes or until chicken cubes are tender.

OR The next day, place casserole dish (with lid on) into microwave oven. Microwave on medium-high for approximately 20 minutes or until chicken cubes are tender.

CHICKEN CASSEROLE

This chicken casserole has a lovely sharp flavor owing to the addition of lemon juice and yogurt. Serve with rice, vegetables, or salad.

PREPARATION TIME: 10 minutes • COOKING TIME: 40 minutes
(20 minutes in microwave)
YIELD: 6 servings

$^2/_3$ cup maize corn flour

1 teaspoon paprika

12 chicken fillets
(skin and fat removed)

2 packets gluten-free soup mix,
vegetable flavor

1$^1/_3$ cups warm water

1 clove garlic, peeled and crushed

1 teaspoon gluten-free
Worcestershire sauce

$^1/_3$ cup white wine

$^2/_3$ cup lemon juice

2 tablespoons low-fat natural yogurt

1 tablespoon finely chopped parsley

1. Preheat oven to 350°F.

2. Prepare a large, flat casserole dish by spraying with cooking spray.

3. Place corn flour into a small bowl and stir in paprika.

4. Toss chicken fillets in seasoned corn flour.

5. Arrange chicken fillets and any remaining seasoned corn flour over base of prepared casserole dish.

6. Combine remaining ingredients in a small bowl and pour over chicken fillets.

7. Cook for approximately 40 minutes or until chicken fillets are tender.

OR Microwave on medium-high for approximately 20 minutes or until chicken fillets are tender.

CHICKEN WITH CHERRY SAUCE

*This is a delicious recipe. The sauce accompanying the chicken
has a sweet and sour flavor. The color presentation is excellent.
It is a good recipe to serve for a dinner party of 6 guests.
Serve with jacket potatoes and side salad.*

PREPARATION TIME: 12 minutes (+ marinate overnight)
COOKING TIME: Approximately 20 minutes
YIELD: 6 servings

Chicken

6 large chicken fillets
(skin and fat removed)

$\frac{1}{3}$ cup gluten-free soy sauce

Freshly ground black pepper

6 thin slices lemon

1 tablespoon olive oil

Cherry Sauce

16 oz can pitted black cherries
(in natural juice)

4 tablespoons white distilled vinegar

8 tablespoons brown sugar

$2\frac{2}{3}$ cups gluten-free chicken or vegetable stock

1 tablespoon finely grated orange rind

1 tablespoon finely grated lemon rind

$1\frac{1}{3}$ cups orange juice (no added sugar)

4 tablespoons lemon juice

4 tablespoons maize corn flour

Chicken

1. Place chicken fillets into a flat dish. Brush both sides of fillets with soy sauce. Pour any remaining sauce over fillets.

2. Sprinkle pepper over fillets, and place a slice of lemon on each fillet. Cover and marinate in refrigerator overnight.

3. The next day, drain chicken fillets and discard marinade.

4. Pour oil into a large nonstick frying pan and heat pan.

5. Place chicken fillets into heated pan. Cook, turning frequently, until chicken fillets are tender.

6. Set chicken fillets aside and keep warm while preparing cherry sauce.

Cherry Sauce

1. Strain cherries and reserve liquid.

2. Place vinegar and brown sugar into a small saucepan. Bring to a boil, stirring constantly until mixture caramelizes. Take care not to burn the mixture.

3. Allow mixture to cool slightly. Stir in stock, rinds, and juices.

4. Place corn flour into a small bowl. Blend with reserved cherry juice.

5. Pour blended corn flour and cherry juice into saucepan. Stir over a gentle heat until sauce boils and thickens.

6. Remove from heat and stir cherries into sauce.

7. Serve hot cherry sauce over chicken fillets and lemon slices.

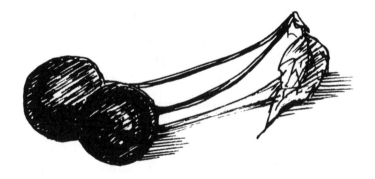

CHICKEN AND PINEAPPLE

This recipe uses pineapple to give a sweet and sour flavor. The chicken is best if marinated overnight to develop the flavor; however, an acceptable flavor can be obtained without marinating. Serve with rice and/or salad.

PREPARATION TIME: 12 minutes (+ marinate overnight)
COOKING TIME: 55 minutes (25 minutes in microwave)
YIELD: 6 servings

2 lbs chicken fillets (skin and fat removed)
3 x 8 oz cans pineapple pieces (in natural juice)
3 tablespoons gluten-free soy sauce
2 tablespoons white distilled vinegar
2 tablespoons brown sugar
1 large onion
$\frac{1}{2}$ red bell pepper
$\frac{1}{2}$ green bell pepper
3 tablespoons maize corn flour
3 tablespoons cold water

1. Prepare a large casserole dish (with lid) by spraying with cooking spray.

2. Cut chicken fillets into small cubes. Place chicken cubes into prepared casserole dish.

3. Add pineapple pieces and juice, soy sauce, vinegar, and brown sugar.

4. Cover and marinate in refrigerator overnight.

5. The next day, peel and slice onion and add to casserole dish.

6. Place casserole dish (with lid on) into a cold oven. Turn oven to 350°F and cook for 40 minutes. Cut peppers into thin strips and stir into casserole dish. Cook for another 15 minutes (with lid off).

OR Place casserole dish into microwave oven. Microwave on high for 20 minutes (with lid on). Cut peppers into thin strips and stir into casserole dish. Microwave on high for another 5 minutes (with lid off).

7. Place corn flour into a small bowl. Blend with water. Stir into casserole.

8. Cook for another 5 minutes or until sauce thickens.

OR Microwave on high for another 2 minutes or until sauce thickens.

COCONUT LIME CHICKEN

PREPARATION TIME: 15 minutes • COOKING TIME: 25 minutes
YIELD: 6–8 servings with salad

1 lb pumpkin

1 lb chicken breast fillets

$\frac{1}{3}$ cup gluten-free corn flour

1 tablespoon olive oil

2 onions

1 tablespoon olive oil, extra

$7\frac{1}{2}$ oz can light coconut milk

1 lime

2 tablespoons finely chopped
fresh coriander

Freshly ground black pepper,
as desired

$1\frac{1}{3}$ cups grated, low-fat
cheddar cheese

2 tablespoons gluten-free
cornflake crumbs

1. Peel and cut pumpkin into $\frac{1}{2}$-inch cubes. Place into a saucepan with a small quantity of water and cook until just tender. Do not overcook. While pumpkin is cooking, prepare chicken.

2. Preheat oven to 350°F.

3. Prepare a large casserole dish by spraying with cooking spray.

4. Cut chicken fillets into approximately $\frac{1}{2}$-inch cubes.

5. Place corn flour into a medium-sized bowl. Toss chicken cubes in corn flour.

6. Pour oil into a frying pan. Add about half the chicken cubes and cook until golden brown. Place into prepared casserole dish. Place remainder of chicken cubes into frying pan. If necessary, add a little more oil. Cook remainder of cubes and place in casserole dish.

7. Peel and finely dice onions. Add extra 1 tablespoon oil to pan. Add onion to pan and sauté until just tender. Do not brown onion. Add to chicken in casserole dish.

8. Strain pumpkin and discard liquid. Place pumpkin into casserole dish.

9. Pour coconut milk into a small bowl.

10. Squeeze lime and stir juice into coconut milk. Stir in coriander and pepper. Pour into casserole dish.

11. Top with grated cheese and cornflake crumbs.

12. Place into a moderate oven and bake for approximately 25 minutes or until golden brown.

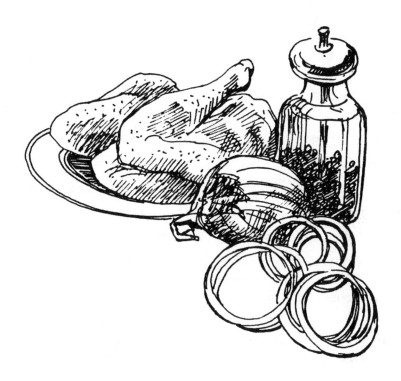

CRANBERRY CITRUS CHICKEN

This chicken has a delicious blend of cranberry sauce and citrus juices.
The citrus juices make the chicken very tender and the flavor is superb.
Serve on a bed of cooked rice.

PREPARATION TIME: 12 minutes (+ marinate overnight)
COOKING TIME: 35 minutes (20 minutes in microwave)
YIELD: 6 servings

2 lbs chicken fillets (skin and fat removed)
2 tablespoons maize corn flour
2 tablespoons water
16 oz jar cranberry sauce (gluten-free)
1 teaspoon finely grated orange rind
$1\frac{1}{3}$ cups orange juice (no added sugar)
Juice of $\frac{1}{2}$ a lemon
1 tablespoon finely chopped fresh ginger
$\frac{2}{3}$ cup white wine
1 teaspoon gluten-free mustard

1. Prepare a 4-pint flat casserole dish (with lid) by spraying with cooking spray.

2. Place chicken fillets over base of prepared casserole dish.

3. Place corn flour into a small bowl. Blend with water.

4. Pour blended corn flour into a large bowl. Mix in remaining ingredients.

5. Pour mixture over chicken fillets.

6. Cover and marinate in refrigerator overnight.

7. The next day, place casserole dish (with lid on) into a cold oven. Turn oven to 350°F and cook for approximately 35 minutes or until chicken fillets are tender, stirring occasionally.

OR The next day, place casserole dish (with lid on) into microwave oven. Microwave on high for approximately 20 minutes or until chicken fillets are tender, stirring occasionally.

SEAFOOD

SALMON PIE

This is a tasty fish pie with a crisp pastry base.
Freshly cooked salmon can be used in place
of canned salmon if desired. Serve with salad.

PREPARATION TIME: 15 minutes • COOKING TIME: 40 minutes
YIELD: 4–6 servings

Pastry

$^2/_3$ cup white rice flour

$^2/_3$ cup gluten-free, plain, all-purpose flour

2 teaspoons gluten-free baking powder

$^2/_3$ cup ground rice

1 tablespoon polenta

6 tablespoons salt-reduced
monounsaturated margarine

Water to moisten dry ingredients
(approx. $^1/_3$ cup)

Filling

16 oz canned pink salmon

$^2/_3$ cup finely chopped celery

$^2/_3$ cup finely chopped shallots

1 medium-sized tomato, diced

$^2/_3$ cup frozen peas

$^2/_3$ cup grated low-fat tasty cheese

1 tablespoon freshly grated
parmesan cheese

Pastry

1. Preheat oven to 400°F.

2. Prepare a 9-inch pie dish by spraying with cooking spray.

3. Sift flours and baking powder into a medium-sized mixing bowl. Stir in ground rice and polenta.

4. Rub margarine into dry ingredients until mixture resembles fine bread crumbs. This process may be done by hand or with the aid of an electric food processor.

5. Stir in sufficient water to mix to a firm dough.

6. Turn dough out onto a lightly floured (gluten-free) board and knead lightly.

7. Gently roll pastry out to approximately $\frac{1}{4}$-inch thickness to fit base and sides of pie dish.

8. Carefully line base and sides of prepared pie dish with pastry.

9. Place pie dish onto a flat oven tray to facilitate handling.

Filling

1. Drain salmon and discard liquid. Lightly flake salmon and remove bones. Place salmon onto pastry in pie dish.

2. Mix celery, shallots, tomato, and peas in a small basin. Spread evenly over salmon.

3. Decorate top of pie with any remaining pastry.

4. Sprinkle cheeses over pie.

5. Place pie into oven and cook for approximately 40 minutes or until lightly golden brown and pastry is cooked.

Tuna Casserole

*There are many variations of a tuna casserole. This recipe
contains no eggs, no gluten products, and uses low-fat cheese.
Freshly cooked tuna can be used in place of canned tuna.*

PREPARATION TIME: 30 minutes • COOKING TIME: 10 minutes
(5 minutes in microwave)

YIELD: 6 servings

$1\frac{2}{3}$ cups basmati rice

4 cups cold water

16 oz canned tuna (no oil, no added salt)

$1\frac{1}{3}$ cups frozen peas

1 large onion, peeled and finely chopped

16 oz canned peeled tomatoes (no added salt)

Approximately 2 cups low-fat milk

2 tablespoons maize corn flour

2 tablespoons finely chopped fresh parsley

$\frac{1}{4}$ teaspoon dried basil leaves

Freshly ground black pepper, as desired

$\frac{2}{3}$ cup grated low-fat cheddar cheese

1 tablespoon freshly grated parmesan cheese

Sprigs of parsley (for garnish)

1. Place rice and water into a large saucepan. Cook over a low heat until rice is tender and water is absorbed.

OR Place rice and water into a medium-sized microwave-safe bowl. Microwave on medium-high for approximately 9 minutes or until rice is tender and water is absorbed.

2. Prepare a 4-pint casserole dish by spraying with cooking spray.

3. Spread cooked rice over base of prepared casserole dish.

4. Drain tuna and reserve liquid. Spread tuna over rice in casserole dish.

5. Spread peas over tuna in casserole dish.

6. Lightly spray a nonstick frying pan with cooking spray. Lightly cook onion and place into casserole dish.

7. Chop tomatoes and spread over ingredients in casserole dish.

8. Pour reserved tuna liquid into a measuring jug. Add milk to make $2\frac{2}{3}$ cups of liquid.

9. Place corn flour into a small saucepan. Add a little liquid and blend well. Gradually stir in remaining liquid. Cook over a low heat until sauce boils and thickens.

OR Place corn flour into a small microwave-safe bowl. Add a little liquid and blend well. Gradually stir in remaining liquid. Microwave on high for 1 minute and stir. Continue to microwave on high, stirring at 40 second intervals, until sauce thickens.

10. Stir chopped parsley, basil, and black pepper into sauce.

11. Pour sauce over casserole, and sprinkle cheeses over sauce.

12. Preheat oven to 350°F. Bake for 10 minutes or until heated through.

OR Microwave on high for 5 minutes or until heated through.

13. Garnish with sprigs of fresh parsley.

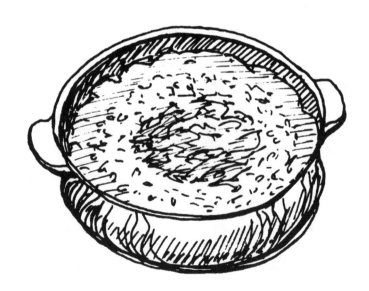

TUNA MORNAY

Pasta and tuna are excellent inclusions in a healthy eating program.

PREPARATION TIME: 15 minutes • COOKING TIME: 30 minutes
(8 minutes in microwave)
YIELD: 4–6 servings

8 oz gluten-free pasta

13$\frac{1}{2}$ oz canned tuna in spring water

3 tablespoons gluten-free corn flour

1$\frac{1}{2}$ pts skim milk

1$\frac{1}{3}$ cups grated low-fat cheddar cheese

2 tablespoons gluten-free crushed cornflakes

$\frac{1}{2}$ teaspoon dried garden herbs of your choice

2 tablespoons finely grated parmesan

1. Preheat oven to 400°F.

2. Prepare a large casserole dish by spraying with cooking spray.

3. Place pasta into boiling water and simmer until just soft. It is important not to overcook pasta. Drain and place into prepared dish.

4. Drain tuna and discard liquid. Spread tuna over pasta.

5. Place corn flour into a medium-sized bowl. Pour in a little milk. Blend until smooth. Pour in remaining milk.

6. Place sauce into a medium-sized saucepan. Cook over a gentle heat stirring continuously until sauce boils and thickens.

OR Place sauce into a microwave-safe bowl. Microwave on high for 1 minute and stir. Continue to microwave on medium high stirring at 1 minute intervals until sauce boils and thickens.

7. Pour sauce over tuna. Top with grated cheese, cornflake crumbs, herbs, and parmesan.

8. Place into a moderately hot oven for approximately 30 minutes, or until heated through and golden brown.

OR Microwave on medium-high for 8 minutes or until heated through.

9. Remove from oven and serve as a main meal with salad.

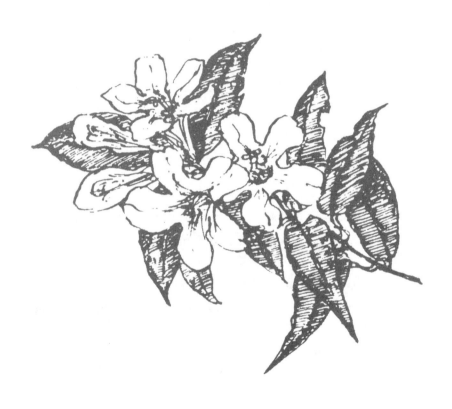

7.

Salads and Vegetables

Salads

Avocado Salad, 94

Cucumber Dressing, 95

Green and Gold Salad, 96

Potato Salad, 97

Potato and Mushroom
Salad, 98

Spinach Salad, 99

Sweet Potato Salad, 100

Tofu Mayonnaise, 101

Vegetables

Curried Lentil Pie, 102

Olive and Fig Tapenade, 103

Potato and Leek Casserole, 104

Potato and Leek Slice, 105

Potato Casserole, 106

Potato Pie, 107

Potato Soy Bake, 108

Pumpkin and Feta
Quiche, 109

Spinach Pie, 110

Spinach Vegetable Rice,
112

Tomato Pie, 114

Vegetable Pie, 116

Vegetable Stir-Fry, 117

Zucchini with Lime
and Garlic, 118

Zucchini Pancakes, 119

SALADS

AVOCADO SALAD

Celery, avocado, apple, and walnuts are combined to make this tasty salad. It is best served immediately after it is prepared.

PREPARATION TIME: 12 minutes

YIELD: 4–6 side salads

$2\frac{2}{3}$ cups shredded lettuce
(of your choice)

$\frac{2}{3}$ cup finely chopped celery

1 avocado

1 apple

2 tablespoons lemon juice

$\frac{2}{3}$ cup chopped walnuts

$\frac{1}{3}$ cup gluten-free French dressing
with garlic (no oil)

1. Place shredded lettuce into a salad serving bowl.

2. Add celery to lettuce.

3. Peel avocado and cut into $\frac{1}{2}$-inch cubes. Place into a small bowl.

4. Peel, core, and finely dice apple and add to avocado.

5. Pour lemon juice over apple and avocado and stir gently. Add to lettuce.

6. Add walnuts to salad.

7. Pour on dressing and toss lightly.

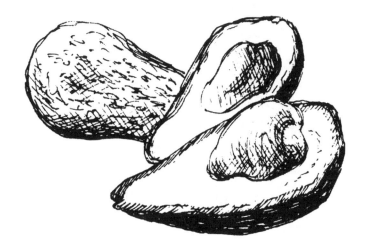

CUCUMBER DRESSING

*This dressing is suitable to serve with salad, meat, or fish as desired.
It is also a suitable accompaniment for sandwich fillings.*

PREPARATION TIME: **5 minutes**

10$\frac{1}{2}$ oz packet tofu (soybean curd)
1 small green-skinned cucumber (skin removed)
$\frac{1}{4}$ teaspoon crushed garlic
$\frac{1}{2}$ teaspoon cracked black peppercorns
1 tablespoon olive oil
1 teaspoon gluten-free prepared mustard

1. Place all the ingredients into the bowl of an electric food processor or blender and blend until smooth.

2. Store in a sealed container and refrigerate until required.

GREEN AND GOLD SALAD

This recipe will appeal to those who like grapefruit. If you do not like the sharpness of grapefruit, you can use extra oranges. If you are not ready to serve this salad immediately, you can seal the avocado, orange, and grapefruit and refrigerate until required.

PREPARATION TIME: **12 minutes**
YIELD: **6 side salads**

Lettuce leaves (of your choice)
2 avocados
2 oranges
1 grapefruit
2 tablespoons olive oil
1 tablespoon white distilled vinegar
1 teaspoon superfine sugar

1. Arrange lettuce leaves in a medium-sized salad bowl.

2. Peel avocados and cut into small cubes. Place into a small bowl.

3. Peel oranges and grapefruit and cut into small cubes. Add to avocado.

4. Mix avocado, orange, and grapefruit together gently. Arrange over lettuce leaves in salad bowl.

5. Mix olive oil, vinegar, and sugar in a small jug and pour over salad.

6. Serve immediately.

POTATO SALAD

Potato salad is usually a family favorite.

PREPARATION TIME: 20 minutes (this allows time to cook potato)

YIELD: 6 servings

4 large potatoes

$\frac{2}{3}$ cup low-fat natural yogurt

1 stick celery, cut into small pieces

2 pickles, cut into small pieces (gluten-free)

6 small pickled onions, cut into small pieces

3 stuffed olives, cut into small pieces

1 tablespoon finely chopped red bell pepper

$\frac{2}{3}$ cup gluten-free herb and green pepper dressing,
or other gluten-free dressing (no oil)

1 tablespoon finely chopped parsley

$\frac{1}{2}$ teaspoon gluten-free mustard

1. Peel potatoes and cut into small cubes.

2. Place potato into a steamer and cook until potato is just tender. Do not overcook or potato cubes will break up.

OR Spread potato over a large, flat microwave-safe plate. Cover with vented plastic wrap. Microwave on high for approximately 7 minutes or until potato is tender.

3. Place potato cubes into a serving dish and allow to cool while preparing yogurt dressing.

4. Mix remaining ingredients together in a small bowl and pour over potato in serving dish just before serving.

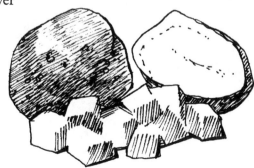

POTATO AND MUSHROOM SALAD

*This salad is suitable for those who like a variation
to ordinary potato salad.*

PREPARATION TIME: 20 minutes (this allows time to cook potato)
YIELD: 4–6 servings as a main meal
or 6–8 as a side salad

6 large potatoes

12 mushrooms

2 sticks celery

$\frac{1}{2}$ cup finely chopped shallots

8 oz ricotta cheese

$\frac{2}{3}$ cup gluten-free French dressing (no oil)

1 teaspoon dried salad herbs

1. Peel potatoes and cut into small cubes.

2. Place potato into a steamer and cook until potato is just tender. Do not overcook or potato cubes will break up.

OR Spread potato over a large, flat microwave-safe plate. Cover with vented plastic wrap. Microwave on high for approximately 10 minutes or until potato is tender.

3. Place potato into a large salad bowl.

4. Wash mushrooms and cut into small cubes. (Skins may be removed if desired). Place into salad bowl.

5. Dice celery and add to salad bowl.

6. Add shallots to salad bowl.

7. Chop cheese and add to salad bowl and toss lightly.

8. Just before serving, pour in dressing, sprinkle with herbs, and toss lightly.

SPINACH SALAD

This very interesting salad is made with uncooked spinach.
It is important to use young, fresh spinach.

PREPARATION TIME: 10 minutes

YIELD: 6 servings

6 young, fresh spinach leaves

2 spring onions

12 small mushrooms

1 tablespoon finely granulated
white sugar

1 tablespoon olive oil

1 tablespoon gluten-free soy sauce

1. Wash and finely shred spinach leaves. Place into a large bowl.

2. Wash onions. Finely slice.

3. Add onion to spinach.

4. Wash mushrooms and cut into thin slices (skins may be removed if desired). Add to spinach.

5. Mix sugar, oil, and soy sauce in a small jug. Pour dressing over spinach and toss well.

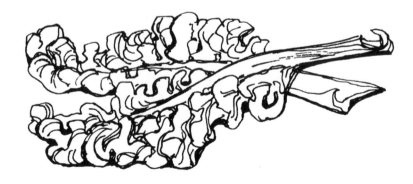

SWEET POTATO SALAD

PREPARATION TIME: 12 minutes • COOKING TIME: 10 minutes
YIELD: 6–8 servings

4 medium sweet potatoes

$\frac{2}{3}$ cup cold water

$\frac{2}{3}$ cup orange juice

2 onions, peeled and finely diced

1 tablespoon olive oil

8 oz diced ham off the bone

4 hard-boiled eggs

4 oz low-fat feta cheese

1 avocado

8 oz sour cream

1 lime

1 teaspoon chopped fresh coriander

1 teaspoon freshly chopped chili, as desired

Lettuce leaves, for serving

1. Peel and finely dice sweet potato. Place into a medium-sized saucepan with water and orange juice. Cook over a gentle heat until just tender. Do not overcook or sweet potato will break up.

2. Strain sweet potato and discard liquid. Place potato into a medium-sized serving bowl.

3. Place onion and oil into a small frying pan. Sauté onion until just soft. Do not brown onion. Add to sweet potato.

4. Place ham onto sweet potato.

5. Peel and chop eggs and add to sweet potato.

6. Chop feta cheese and add to bowl.

7. Peel and dice avocado. Add to sweet potato.

8. Place sour cream into a small bowl. Squeeze lime and stir juice into sour cream. Stir coriander and chili into sour cream.

9. When required, place portions of salad over lettuce leaves. Pour sour cream dressing over salad.

TOFU MAYONNAISE

*This is an alternative mayonnaise to serve
with salad or fish, as desired.*

PREPARATION TIME: **6 minutes**

10½ oz package tofu (soybean curd)

⅔ cup chopped shallots

1 tablespoon honey

½ teaspoon crushed garlic

½ teaspoon cracked black peppercorns

1 teaspoon gluten-free mustard

Juice of 1 lemon

1 tablespoon peanut oil

1. Place all the ingredients into the bowl of an electric food processor or blender. Blend until smooth (or mix together by hand).

2. Store in a sealed container and refrigerate until required.

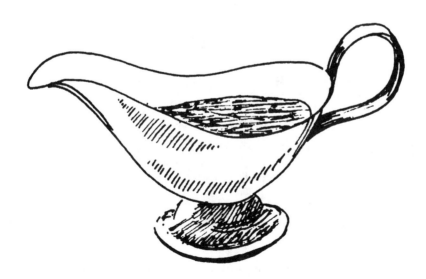

VEGETABLES

CURRIED LENTIL PIE

This recipe was designed for those who have a very low income and find it difficult to provide nutritious family meals.

PREPARATION TIME: **25 minutes** • COOKING TIME: **20 minutes**
(**10 minutes in microwave**)
YIELD: **6 servings**

13 oz whole green lentils

3 medium-sized potatoes

1 tablespoon low-fat milk

1 onion, peeled and finely diced

$\frac{1}{2}$ teaspoon dried minced garlic

2 tablespoons gluten-free Worcestershire sauce

2 teaspoons concentrated gluten-free vegetable stock

1 teaspoon gluten-free curry powder

1$\frac{1}{3}$ cups gluten-free bread crumbs

$\frac{1}{3}$ cup grated low-fat cheddar cheese

1 carrot, peeled and finely grated

1. Place lentils into a large bowl. Cover with warm water and seal. When cool, refrigerate overnight.

2. The next day, strain and thoroughly rinse lentils.

3. Preheat oven to 350°F.

4. Prepare a large casserole dish by spraying with cooking spray.

5. Peel and dice potatoes. Place into a large saucepan with a small amount of water. Bring to a boil and cook with the lid on until potato is tender.

6. Strain potato and mash with milk. Spread mashed potato over base of prepared casserole dish.

7. Place lentils into a saucepan with $2\frac{2}{3}$ cups boiling water. Cook for 10 minutes with lid off.

8. Add onion to saucepan. Cook with lid on until lentils are tender.

9. Strain lentils and onion. Place lentils and onion into a medium-sized bowl. Stir in garlic, Worcestershire sauce, vegetable stock, and curry. Spread seasoned lentils over mashed potato.

10. Mix bread crumbs and cheese in a small bowl. Sprinkle over lentils.

11. Arrange a ring of grated carrot around outer edge of pie.

12. Place pie into oven and cook for approximately 20 minutes or until heated through and golden brown on top.

OR Microwave on high for approximately 10 minutes or until heated through.

OLIVE AND FIG TAPENADE

This paste can be used to serve with cooked meat or as an accompaniment to focaccia or a cheese platter.

PREPARATION TIME: 10 minutes

$1\frac{1}{3}$ cups dried figs

$1\frac{1}{3}$ cups black olives, pitted

6 anchovy fillets, drained and rinsed

1 tablespoon capers, drained

5 tablespoons lemon juice

2 sprigs mint

Freshly ground black pepper,
as desired

$1\frac{1}{3}$ cups olive oil

1. Place all the ingredients except the oil into the bowl of an electric blender. Blend until smooth.

2. Very slowly trickle oil into blender and blend until smooth.

3. Seal in a container and store in the refrigerator until required.

POTATO AND LEEK CASSEROLE

This casserole will please those who like the combination of potato and leek.

PREPARATION TIME: 20 minutes • COOKING TIME: 20 minutes
(10 minutes in microwave)
YIELD: 6 servings

6 large potatoes
3 tablespoons potato flour
1 pint carton cultured buttermilk
$\frac{1}{2}$ leek, cut into thin slices
$\frac{2}{3}$ cup grated low-fat tasty cheese
2 tablespoons freshly grated parmesan cheese

1. Preheat oven to 350°F.

2. Prepare a large, flat casserole dish by spraying with cooking spray.

3. Peel potatoes and cut into $\frac{1}{2}$-inch slices.

4. Place potato into a steamer and cook until potato is just tender. Do not overcook or potato slices will break up.

OR Spread potato over a large, flat microwave-safe plate. Cover with vented plastic wrap. Microwave on high for approximately 10 minutes or until potato is tender.

5. Place potato flour into a medium-sized saucepan. Stir in a little buttermilk and blend well. Gradually stir in remaining buttermilk. Cook over a low heat, stirring continuously until sauce boils and thickens.

OR Place potato flour into a 2 pint microwave-safe jug. Stir in a little buttermilk and blend well. Gradually stir in remaining buttermilk. Microwave on high for 40 seconds and stir. Continue to microwave on high, stirring at 40 second intervals, until sauce thickens.

6. Spread half the cooked potato slices over base of prepared casserole dish. Spread leek slices over potato, and pour half the sauce over leek slices. Then add remaining potato slices, and pour on remaining sauce.

7. Sprinkle with grated tasty cheese. Top with parmesan cheese.

8. Place casserole into oven and cook for approximately 20 minutes or until heated through.

OR Microwave on high for about 10 minutes or until heated through.

POTATO AND LEEK SLICE

This is a delicious combination of vegetables baked with egg and cheese.
It can be served hot or cold.

PREPARATION TIME: 15 minutes • COOKING TIME: 40 minutes
YIELD: 6 servings

2 medium-sized potatoes

$\frac{1}{2}$ a small butternut pumpkin

1 large carrot

1 leek

3 eggs

$2\frac{2}{3}$ cups gluten-free, plain,
all-purpose flour

$\frac{2}{3}$ cup olive oil

$1\frac{1}{3}$ cups grated low-fat cheddar cheese

2 tablespoons freshly grated parmesan cheese

Freshly ground black pepper, as desired

1. Preheat oven to 350°F.

2. Prepare a 10-inch square pan by spraying with cooking spray. Line base of pan with baking paper.

3. Peel and grate potato, pumpkin, and carrot.

4. Wash and finely chop white part of leek. Place into a flat microwave-proof dish and microwave on high for 1 minute. Stir and microwave on high for another 1 minute.

5. Place vegetables into a large bowl.

6. Lightly beat eggs and pour into vegetables.

7. Stir in flour, oil, grated cheese, parmesan cheese, and pepper. Pour into prepared pan.

8. Place into a moderate oven and bake for approximately 40 minutes or until set in the center.

9. When cooked, remove from oven and allow to stand for 10 minutes before cutting into slices for serving.

POTATO CASSEROLE

This casserole is very easy to prepare.

PREPARATION TIME: 20 minutes (includes time to cook potato)
COOKING TIME: 12 minutes (5 minutes in microwave)
YIELD: 6 servings

6 medium-sized potatoes

1 tablespoon salt-reduced
monounsaturated margarine

Freshly ground black pepper,
as desired

$1\frac{1}{3}$ cups chopped shallots

1 cup light sour cream

$\frac{2}{3}$ cup grated low-fat cheese

1 tablespoon freshly grated
parmesan cheese

1. Preheat oven to 425°F.

2. Prepare a large, flat casserole dish by spraying with cooking spray.

3. Peel and dice potatoes.

4. Place potato into a steamer and cook until potato is tender.

OR Spread potato over a large, flat microwave-safe plate. Cover with vented plastic wrap. Microwave on high for approximately 10 minutes or until potato is tender.

5. Mash potato with margarine and pepper. Add shallots and sour cream to potato and mix well.

6. Spread potato mixture over base of prepared dish. Sprinkle with cheeses.

7. Place casserole into oven and cook for approximately 12 minutes or until heated through and cheese is golden brown.

OR Microwave on high for approximately 5 minutes or until heated through.

POTATO PIE

Serve this dish as desired with meat or fish.

PREPARATION TIME: 12 minutes • COOKING TIME: 1 hour
(20 minutes in microwave)
YIELD: 6 servings

6 medium-to-large potatoes

1 small onion

$2/3$ cup low-fat natural yogurt

$1\frac{1}{3}$ cups low-fat evaporated milk

1 package gluten-free soup mix,
vegetable flavor

8 oz ricotta cheese

Freshly ground black pepper, as desired

$2/3$ cup gluten-free bread crumbs

$2/3$ cup grated low-fat tasty cheese

1 tablespoon finely chopped parsley
(for garnish)

1. Preheat oven to 350°F.

2. Prepare a large, flat ovenproof dish by spraying with cooking spray.

3. Peel potatoes and slice thinly.

4. Arrange potato slices over base of prepared dish.

5. Peel and finely chop onion and sprinkle over potato.

6. Mix yogurt, evaporated milk, soup mix, ricotta cheese, and pepper in a medium-sized bowl. Pour over potato and onion in dish.

7. Sprinkle bread crumbs and cheese over pie.

8. Place pie into oven and cook for approximately 1 hour or until potato is tender.

OR Microwave on high for approximately 20 minutes or until potato is tender.

9. Garnish with chopped parsley.

POTATO SOY BAKE

This recipe is for those who like soybeans.

PREPARATION TIME: 20 minutes (including time for potatoes to cook)
COOKING TIME: 20 minutes (10 minutes in microwave)
YIELD: 4–6 servings

6 medium-sized potatoes
1 teaspoon gluten-free mustard
1 tablespoon gluten-free soy drink
16 oz can soybeans (in tomato sauce, if available)
2 sticks celery, finely chopped
$\frac{1}{2}$ red bell pepper, finely chopped
$1\frac{1}{3}$ cups frozen peas
1 onion, peeled and finely chopped
$\frac{2}{3}$ cup gluten-free bread crumbs
$\frac{2}{3}$ cup grated low-fat tasty cheese
1 tablespoon freshly grated parmesan cheese

1. Preheat oven to 350°F.

2. Prepare a 4-pint casserole dish by spraying with cooking spray.

3. Peel and dice potatoes.

4. Place potato into a steamer and cook until potato is tender.

OR Spread potato over a large, flat microwave-safe plate. Cover with vented plastic wrap. Microwave on high for approximately 10 minutes or until potato is tender.

5. Mash potato with mustard and soy drink.

6. Line base and sides of casserole dish with half of the mashed potato.

7. Place soybeans onto potato in casserole dish.

8. Spread celery, pepper, peas, and onion over potato.

9. Top with remaining mashed potato.

10. Sprinkle bread crumbs and cheeses over potato.

11. Place dish into oven and cook for approximately 20 minutes or until heated through and golden brown.

OR Microwave on high for about 10 minutes or until heated through.

PUMPKIN AND FETA QUICHE

The flavor of this quiche is developed in the baking
of the pumpkin prior to making the quiche.

PREPARATION TIME: 30 minutes (includes cooking time for pumpkin)
COOKING TIME: 40 minutes
YIELD: 6 servings

$\frac{1}{2}$ butternut pumpkin

1 teaspoon cracked black pepper

2 teaspoons garlic powder

1 teaspoon dried basil

1 teaspoon dried rosemary

3 tablespoons olive oil

Juice of 1 lemon

$3\frac{1}{2}$ oz crumbled feta

1 onion, peeled and finely chopped

1 tablespoon freshly chopped parsley

$\frac{2}{3}$ cup gluten-free self-raising flour

$\frac{2}{3}$ cup light sour cream

$\frac{2}{3}$ cup low-fat milk

4 eggs

Salt and freshly ground black pepper, as desired

$1\frac{1}{3}$ cups grated low-fat cheddar cheese

1. Preheat oven to 350°F.

2. Prepare a 9-inch quiche dish by spraying with cooking spray.

3. Peel and thinly slice pumpkin. Place over base of prepared dish.

4. Mix pepper, garlic, basil, and rosemary and sprinkle over pumpkin.

5. Mix oil and lemon juice and pour over pumpkin.

6. Place into a moderate oven and bake for 20 minutes or until pumpkin is cooked.

7. When cooked, remove from oven and place dish onto a heatproof board.

8. Spread feta over pumpkin.

9. Place onion, parsley, gluten-free flour, sour cream, milk, eggs, salt, and pepper into the bowl of an electric food processor. Blend well. Pour into quiche dish.

10. Sprinkle with grated cheese.

11. Place into a moderate oven and bake for approximately 40 minutes or until cooked when tested in the center of the quiche.

12. When cooked, remove from oven and allow to stand for 5 minutes. Serve warm or cold with salad as desired.

SPINACH PIE

This lovely spinach pie can be served hot or cold.

PREPARATION TIME: 25 minutes • COOKING TIME: 45 minutes
YIELD: 6–8 servings

Filling
6 fresh spinach leaves

2 eggs

1$\frac{1}{3}$ cups low-fat milk

2 tablespoons finely chopped parsley

$\frac{1}{2}$ teaspoon dried basil

1 teaspoon dried salad herbs

Pastry
1$\frac{1}{3}$ cups gluten-free, plain, all-purpose flour

$\frac{2}{3}$ cup brown rice flour

$\frac{1}{3}$ cup soy flour

2 teaspoons gluten-free baking powder

$\frac{1}{3}$ cup ground rice

3 tablespoons salt-reduced
monounsaturated margarine

Water to moisten dry ingredients (approx. $\frac{1}{3}$ cup)

1$\frac{1}{3}$ cups grated low-fat tasty cheese

2 tablespoons freshly grated parmesan cheese

Filling

1. Wash and finely chop spinach leaves.

2. Place spinach leaves into a steamer and lightly steam with lid on.

3. Place spinach leaves into a medium-sized mixing bowl.

4. Break eggs into a small bowl and lightly beat. Add milk and herbs and mix well. Pour into bowl with spinach and mix well.

Pastry

1. Preheat oven to 400°F.

2. Prepare a 9-inch pie dish by spraying with cooking spray.

3. Sift flours and baking powder into a medium-sized mixing bowl. Stir in ground rice.

4. Rub margarine into dry ingredients until mixture resembles fine bread crumbs. This process may be done by hand or with the aid of an electric food processor.

5. Stir in sufficient water to mix to a firm dough.

6. Turn dough out onto a lightly floured (gluten-free) board and knead lightly.

7. Gently roll pastry to $\frac{1}{4}$-inch thickness to fit base and sides of pie dish.

8. Carefully line prepared pie dish with rolled out pastry.

9. Pour filling into prepared pastry case.

10. Decorate top of pie with any remaining pastry. Sprinkle cheeses over pie.

11. Place pie into oven and cook for approximately 45 minutes or until set in the center when tested.

Spinach Vegetable Rice

This is a tasty vegetarian recipe.

PREPARATION TIME: 30 minutes (allow for time to cook rice
and to bake vegetables) • COOKING TIME: 20 minutes
(8 minutes in microwave)
YIELD: 4 servings

1⅓ cups diced sweet potato

1⅓ cups diced pumpkin

2 tablespoons olive oil

1 clove garlic, peeled and crushed

Cracked black pepper, as desired

2⅔ cups cooked basmati rice

8 oz frozen spinach

2 tablespoons butter or salt-reduced
monounsaturated margarine

2 tablespoons gluten-free, plain,
all-purpose flour

2⅔ cups light milk

14 oz smooth ricotta

2 eggs, well beaten

Ground pepper, as desired

1 cup grated cheddar cheese

1. Preheat oven to 400°F.

2. Prepare an 8-inch round deep casserole dish by spraying with cooking spray.

3. Place sweet potato and pumpkin onto a flat baking dish. Spray well with cooking spray.

4. Pour oil over vegetables.

5. Sprinkle with crushed garlic and cracked pepper.

6. Place into a moderately hot oven and bake until golden brown and vegetables are cooked.

7. Place into prepared casserole dish.

8. Top with rice and spinach.

9. Prepare a sauce by placing butter into a small saucepan and melting over a gentle heat. Remove from heat. Stir in gluten-free flour. Return to heat and cook for 1 minute. Remove from heat. Gradually stir in milk. Return to heat and cook stirring continuously until sauce boils and thickens.

OR Prepare a sauce by placing butter into a small microwave-safe bowl. Microwave on high for 20 seconds. Stir in gluten-free flour. Microwave on medium-high for 30 seconds. Gradually stir in milk. Microwave on medium-high for 1 minute and stir. Continue to microwave on medium-high, stirring at 1 minute intervals until sauce boils and thickens.

10. Stir in ricotta, egg, and ground pepper. Pour sauce over vegetables.

11. Sprinkle with grated cheese.

12. Place into a moderately hot oven and bake for approximately 20 minutes or until golden brown and heated through.

OR Microwave for approximately 8 minutes until heated through.

13. Serve hot or cold as desired.

TOMATO PIE

This savory pie is for those who like a vegetable pie.

PREPARATION TIME: 20 minutes • COOKING TIME: 30 minutes
YIELD: 4–6 servings

Pastry

1²⁄₃ cups gluten-free, plain,
all-purpose flour

²⁄₃ cup white rice flour

¹⁄₃ cup brown rice flour

2 teaspoons gluten-free baking powder

4 tablespoons salt-reduced
monounsaturated margarine

3¹⁄₂ fl oz water (approx.)

Filling

3 tomatoes

¹⁄₃ cup finely chopped celery

²⁄₃ cup finely grated carrot

1 tablespoon finely chopped parsley

¹⁄₃ cup grated apple

1 teaspoon finely grated lemon rind

¹⁄₄ teaspoon dried mixed herbs

²⁄₃ cup gluten-free bread crumbs

²⁄₃ cup grated low-fat tasty cheese

1 tablespoon freshly grated
parmesan cheese

Pastry

1. Preheat oven to 400°F.

2. Prepare a 9-inch pie plate by spraying with cooking spray.

3. Sift gluten-free flour, rice flour, and baking powder into a medium-sized mixing bowl.

4. Rub margarine into sifted dry ingredients until mixture resembles fine bread crumbs. This process may be done by hand or with the aid of an electric food processor.

5. Stir in sufficient water to mix to a firm dough.

6. Turn dough out onto a lightly floured (gluten-free) board and knead lightly.

7. Gently roll pastry to approximately $\frac{1}{4}$-inch thickness to fit base and sides of pie plate.

8. Carefully line prepared pie plate with pastry.

Filling

1. Place tomatoes into boiling water and leave for 1 minute. Remove skins.

2. Cut tomatoes into $\frac{1}{2}$-inch slices and arrange over pastry.

3. Spread celery, carrot, parsley, apple, and lemon rind over tomato.

4. Decorate top of pie with any remaining pastry.

5. Mix herbs, bread crumbs, and cheeses in a small bowl. Sprinkle over pie.

6. Place pie into oven and cook for approximately 30 minutes or until golden brown and cooked.

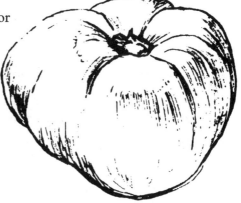

VEGETABLE PIE

This is another tasty vegetarian recipe.

PREPARATION TIME: 15 minutes • COOKING TIME: 30 minutes
(8 minutes in microwave)
YIELD: 4–6 servings

4 cups grated vegetable of your choice
(sweet potato, eggplant, carrot, pumpkin,
potato, onion, and/or cauliflower)

1 clove garlic, peeled and crushed

2 eggs, well beaten

Cracked black pepper, as desired

1 tablespoon chili sauce, as desired

1 tablespoon gluten-free curry paste,
as desired

8 oz tub smooth feta with pepper and herbs

2 tablespoons gluten-free, plain,
all-purpose flour

1 cup grated light cheddar cheese

2 tablespoons grated parmesan cheese

1. Preheat oven to 400°F.

2. Prepare a 9-inch round deep pie dish by spraying with cooking spray.

3. Place all the ingredients except cheddar cheese and parmesan into a large mixing bowl and stir to combine. Spread into prepared pie dish.

4. Sprinkle pie with cheeses.

5. Place into a moderately hot oven and bake for approximately 30 minutes or until firm to touch.

OR Microwave on medium-high for 8 minutes or until firm to touch.

6. Serve hot or cold as desired.

Vegetable Stir-Fry

Crisp and crunchy vegetables are one of my favorite foods.
This recipe can be cooked in a wok or large nonstick frying pan.
Serve on a bed of rice and/or with salad.

PREPARATION TIME: 20 minutes • COOKING TIME: 10 minutes
YIELD: 6 servings

4 oz snow peas

2 teaspoons olive oil

4 oz almond slivers

1 clove garlic, peeled and crushed

2 teaspoons finely chopped fresh ginger

3 large onions, peeled and thickly sliced

1 red bell pepper, seeded and cut into thin strips

8 oz sliced mushrooms

$1\frac{1}{3}$ cups thinly sliced fresh young beans

1 tablespoon maize corn flour

1 cup gluten-free vegetable stock

1 tablespoon gluten-free soy sauce

1 tablespoon gluten-free black bean sauce

1. Remove tops and tails from snow peas and cut into $\frac{1}{2}$-inch pieces.

2. Heat oil in wok.

3. Add almonds and stir until golden brown. Remove almonds from wok and set aside.

4. Add garlic, ginger, and onion to wok and stir until onion softens.

5. Add snow peas, pepper, mushrooms, and beans and stir for 1 minute.

6. Return almonds to wok.

7. Place corn flour into a small bowl. Add a little vegetable stock and blend well. Gradually stir in remaining vegetable stock, soy sauce, and black bean sauce.

8. Pour into wok and stir until sauce thickens.

ZUCCHINI WITH LIME
AND GARLIC

PREPARATION TIME: **8 minutes** • COOKING TIME: **10 minutes**

YIELD: **4 servings as a side dish**

2 tablespoons olive oil

1 onion, peeled and finely chopped

1 clove garlic, peeled and crushed

4 medium-sized zucchini,
cut into $\frac{1}{2}$-inch cubes

1 teaspoon freshly chopped coriander

$\frac{1}{2}$ teaspoon finely grated rind from lime

2 tablespoons lime juice

1. Pour oil into frying pan. Gently heat.

2. Place onion into pan and cook until browned.

3. Add garlic and stir well.

4. Add zucchini. Cover and cook for approximately 5 minutes or until zucchini is just cooked.

5. Add coriander, lime rind and juice. Stir over a gentle heat for 2 minutes.

6. Remove from heat and allow to stand for 5 minutes before serving. Serve hot or cold as desired.

ZUCCHINI PANCAKES

These pancakes can be eaten as a meat substitute
or as a savory snack. Serve warm.

PREPARATION TIME: 20 minutes (includes time to cook pancakes)
YIELD: Approximately 20 pancakes

A little oil to grease pan

$2\frac{2}{3}$ cups grated zucchini

$1\frac{1}{3}$ cups ricotta cheese

1 tablespoon finely chopped mint

$\frac{2}{3}$ cup white rice flour

$\frac{2}{3}$ cup gluten-free, plain,
all-purpose flour

1 teaspoon baking soda

Freshly ground black pepper,
as desired

1 cup cultured buttermilk

$\frac{1}{3}$ cup finely chopped shallots

$\frac{1}{4}$ teaspoon dried basil

$\frac{1}{4}$ teaspoon crushed garlic

1. Heat an electric skillet to 340°F. Lightly oil skillet.

2. Place ingredients into a medium-sized mixing bowl and mix well.

3. Place tablespoons of mixture into heated skillet.

4. Cook on one side until mixture is set on the surface. Turn and cook on reverse side until golden brown and cooked.

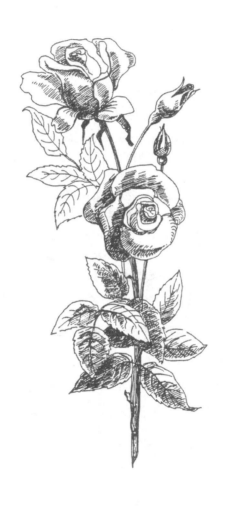

8.

Desserts

Apple Crunch, 122

Almond Halva, 123

Baked Blueberry Cheesecake, 125

Chocolate Sauce Pudding, 127

*Coconut Rice with
Peach-Mango Purée, 128*

Custard, 129

Custard Pie, 130

Fruit in Grape Juice, 131

Fruit Platter with Berry Sauce, 132

Golden Syrup Dumplings, 133

Lemon Meringue Pie, 134

Melon with Cream Cheese, 136

Rhubarb and Strawberry Crumble, 137

*Sticky Date Pudding with
Butterscotch Sauce, 138*

Treacle Tart, 140

Tropical Trifle, 142

APPLE CRUNCH

This recipe is very easy to prepare. It must be made within a couple
of hours of serving or the bread crumbs will go soft. Serve hot
or cold as desired. Serve with custard (see recipe page 129).

PREPARATION TIME: 30 minutes
(allows time to cook apples and crunch)
YIELD: 6 servings

6 large green cooking apples

$\frac{1}{3}$ cup water

Sugar, as desired

$\frac{1}{3}$ cup salt-reduced
monounsaturated margarine

$1\frac{1}{3}$ cup gluten-free bread crumbs

$\frac{1}{3}$ cup almond slivers

$\frac{1}{3}$ cup finely granulated white sugar

$\frac{1}{2}$ teaspoon vanilla extract

1. Prepare an 8-inch round serving dish by spraying with cooking spray.

2. Peel, core, and roughly chop apples. Place into a medium-sized sauce-pan and cook in water with lid on over a low heat until soft. Rub through a sieve or food mill and add sugar (as desired). Set aside.

3. Melt margarine in a frying pan (preferably nonstick).

4. Add bread crumbs, almonds, and sugar. Cook, stirring continuously, until just turning brown. Remove from heat and stir in vanilla.

5. Arrange alternate layers of bread-crumb mixture and apple purée in serving dish, beginning and ending with bread crumbs.

ALMOND HALVA

Halva is a traditional Greek syrup cake. It is usually made with semolina, which is a finely ground cereal made from wheat. In this recipe the semolina is substituted with polenta. Halva may be served hot or cold as desired. As it is very moist, it is best kept in the refrigerator.

PREPARATION TIME: 20 minutes • COOKING TIME: 60 minutes

Cake

$\frac{1}{2}$ cup butter or salt-reduced monounsaturated margarine

2 cups sugar

$\frac{1}{2}$ teaspoon vanilla extract

2 eggs

$1\frac{1}{3}$ cups polenta

$1\frac{1}{3}$ cups ground almonds

1 teaspoon gluten-free baking powder

1 teaspoon finely grated orange rind

3 tablespoons orange juice

Orange Syrup

$1\frac{1}{3}$ cups orange juice

$\frac{2}{3}$ cup sugar

2 tablespoons brandy

1. Preheat oven to 350°F.

2. Prepare a deep 8-inch square cake pan by spraying with cooking spray. Line base of pan with baking paper.

3. Cream butter, sugar, and vanilla and beat well.

4. Lightly beat eggs and gradually add to creamed mixture.

5. Stir in polenta, ground almonds, baking powder, grated orange rind, and juice. Beat well. Spread into prepared pan.

6. Place into a moderate oven and bake for approximately 50 minutes or until very pale golden brown and set when tested.

7. While cake is cooking, combine orange juice and sugar in a medium-sized saucepan. Bring to a boil, stirring constantly to dissolve sugar. Once boiling, do not continue to stir. Boil to reduce syrup and slightly thicken. Remove from heat and stir in brandy.

8. When cake is cooked, remove from oven and leave in pan. Leave the oven on.

9. Pour half the orange syrup over the cake. Allow to stand for 5 minutes. Return to oven and bake for another 5 minutes.

10. Remove cake from oven and pour remaining syrup over cake. Return to oven and bake for another 5 minutes. Remove from oven and allow to cool in pan.

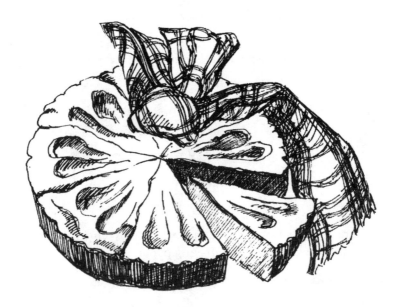

Baked Blueberry Cheesecake

If a plain cheesecake is desired, the blueberries can be omitted.
Cheesecake will keep well in the refrigerator for a few days.
A pastry base can be substituted for the cookie base if desired
(see the recipe for Lemon Meringue Pie on page 134).

PREPARATION TIME: 20 minutes • COOKING TIME: 40 minutes
YIELD: 8 servings

5 oz plain sweet gluten-free cookies

$\frac{1}{2}$ cup butter or salt-reduced
monounsaturated margarine

2 oz ground almonds

$\frac{1}{2}$ teaspoon vanilla extract

7 oz frozen blueberries

$\frac{2}{3}$ cup almond flakes

4 tablespoons cultured butter or salt-reduced
monounsaturated margarine, melted

2 oz gluten-free corn flour

4 eggs

1 lb smooth ricotta

8 oz package cream cheese

Finely grated rind and juice of 1 lemon

5 oz pure icing sugar

$1\frac{1}{4}$ cup light cream

A few drops of almond extract

$\frac{1}{2}$ teaspoon vanilla extract, extra

A little extra pure icing sugar
to dust top of cheesecake for serving

1. Preheat oven to 350°F.

2. Prepare a 9-inch deep, round pie dish by spraying with cooking spray.

3. Crush cookies into fine crumbs. Place into a mixing bowl.

4. Melt butter and pour into cookie crumbs. Add ground almonds and vanilla and mix well. Press into base and sides of prepared dish. It may be helpful to use the back of a large metal spoon to press down the cookie base. Refrigerate while preparing cheesecake filling.

5. Place blueberries on cookie base in dish.

6. Sprinkle almond flakes over blueberries.

7. Place melted butter, corn flour, eggs, ricotta, cream cheese, lemon rind and juice, pure icing sugar, cream, almond extract, and extra vanilla extract into the bowl of an electric blender and blend well. Pour over blueberries in dish.

8. Place into a moderate oven and bake for approximately 40 minutes or until set in the center when tested.

9. When cooked, remove from oven and allow to cool completely before serving.

10. Just before serving, dust with a little extra pure icing sugar.

CHOCOLATE SAUCE PUDDING

*My friend Denise asked me to include a gluten-free chocolate sauce
pudding in this book. This dessert is delicious served hot or cold with
cream, gluten-free ice cream, or custard (see recipe page 129), as desired.*

PREPARATION TIME: 15 minutes • COOKING TIME: 20 minutes
(8 minutes in microwave)
YIELD: 6 servings

$1\frac{1}{3}$ cups gluten-free self-raising flour

2 tablespoons cocoa

1 cup finely granulated white sugar

1 cup milk

1 teaspoon vanilla extract

4 tablespoons butter or salt-reduced
monounsaturated margarine, softened

1 tablespoon cocoa, extra

$\frac{1}{2}$ cup brown sugar

$1\frac{2}{3}$ cups fresh black coffee (for best flavor
use fresh strongly brewed coffee, or make by using
$1\frac{1}{2}$ teaspoons instant coffee in boiling water)

1. Preheat oven to 350°F.

2. Prepare a medium-sized casserole dish by spraying with cooking spray.

3. Sift gluten-free flour and cocoa into a medium-sized mixing bowl. Stir in sugar.

4. Pour in milk and vanilla and stir.

5. Stir in butter. (Butter or margarine must be very soft. It can be softened in the microwave if necessary.)

6. Beat for 2 minutes using a handheld electric mixer until ingredients are well combined. (Beat with a wooden spoon if an electric mixer is not available.)

7. Pour into prepared dish.

8. Place the extra 1 tablespoon cocoa into a small mixing bowl. Stir in brown sugar. Sprinkle over mixture.

9. Carefully pour hot coffee over mixture.

10. Place into a moderate oven and cook for approximately 20 minutes or until cake mixture is cooked when tested.

OR Microwave on high for approximately 8 minutes or until cake mixture is cooked when tested.

11. Allow to stand for 5 minutes before serving.

COCONUT RICE WITH PEACH-MANGO PURÉE

PREPARATION AND COOKING TIME: 40 minutes (25 minutes in microwave)
YIELD: 6 servings

1 1/3 cups basmati rice
2 2/3 cups water
2 2/3 cups low-fat milk
14 oz can light coconut milk
2/3 cup sugar
2 tablespoons honey
1/2 teaspoon vanilla extract
26 oz can peach slices in mango juice

1. Place the rice and water into a saucepan. Bring to a boil. Reduce heat and cook for approximately 15 minutes or until rice is soft.

OR Place the rice and water into a microwave rice cooker. Microwave on high for 2 minutes. Microwave on medium-low until rice is soft. This will be approximately 12 minutes.

2. Remove from heat. Stir in milk. Return to heat and cook for approximately 20 minutes or until liquid has been absorbed by rice.

OR Stir in milk. Microwave on medium-low for approximately 10 minutes or until all liquid is absorbed.

3. When cooked, stir in coconut milk, sugar, honey, and vanilla. Place into a serving bowl.

4. To make the purée, place peach slices in mango juice into the bowl of an electric blender. Blend until smooth.

5. Pour purée over rice for serving.

CUSTARD

PREPARATION TIME: **5 minutes** • COOKING TIME: **7 minutes**
(5 minutes in microwave)
YIELD: **4–6 servings**

2 tablespoons gluten-free corn flour

1 pint low-fat milk

1 egg, lightly beaten

2 tablespoons light cream

3 tablespoons sugar

$\frac{1}{2}$ teaspoon vanilla extract

1. Place corn flour into a small bowl. Blend with a little of the milk. Stir in remainder of milk.

2. Add egg and cream and whisk well.

3. Pour into a small saucepan. Stir constantly over a low heat until custard thickens. DO NOT BOIL, or custard may curdle.

OR Pour into a small microwave-safe bowl. Microwave on medium for 1 minute and stir. Continue to microwave on medium-low, stirring at 1 minute intervals until custard thickens. DO NOT BOIL, or custard may curdle.

4. Stir in sugar and vanilla.

5. Serve hot or cold as desired.

Variation—Almond Custard:
When custard is cooked, add $3\frac{1}{2}$ oz ground almonds and a couple of drops of almond extract.

CUSTARD PIE

*This is a quick-mix recipe that is very easy to prepare. It can be cooked
in a foil tray and easily transported. The pie will have a firm base
representing a pastry base. It is best made the day before it is required.
It is not suitable for freezing.*

PREPARATION TIME: 5 minutes • COOKING TIME: 35 minutes
(10 minutes in microwave)

YIELD: 6 servings

1 tablespoon butter or salt-reduced
monounsaturated margarine, softened

$^2/_3$ cup brown sugar

1 tablespoon potato flour

4 oz cream cheese

3 eggs

$2^2/_3$ cups milk

$^1/_2$ teaspoon vanilla extract

Nutmeg (to sprinkle on top)

1. Preheat oven to 325°F.

2. Prepare a 9-inch round pie dish by spraying with cooking spray.

3. Place all the ingredients except nutmeg into a blender. Blend until
   smooth. (Ingredients can be beaten well using a handheld mixer, or
   beaten with a wooden spoon.)

4. Pour into prepared dish.

5. Place dish into a larger ovenproof dish. Pour enough cold water into the
   larger dish to go about halfway up the outside of the pie dish.

6. Sprinkle top of custard pie with nutmeg.

7. Place into a moderately slow oven and bake for approximately 35 minutes or until custard is set in the center when tested with the point of a
   sharp knife. When cooked, carefully remove from oven. Remove pie
   from dish of hot water and allow to cool.

OR Microwave on medium-high for about 10 minutes or until custard is
   set in the center when tested with the point of a sharp knife. When pie
   is cooked, carefully remove from dish of hot water and allow to cool.

8. Refrigerate before serving.

FRUIT IN GRAPE JUICE

This is a very lovely dessert. It is just good wholesome fruit in fruit juices.
Serve hot or cold as desired.

PREPARATION TIME: 15 minutes (+ overnight soaking)
COOKING TIME: 30 minutes (20 minutes in microwave)
YIELD: 6 servings

$\frac{2}{3}$ cup natural golden raisins
(sultanas)

$\frac{2}{3}$ cup natural currants

$\frac{2}{3}$ cup chopped dates

1 tablespoon mixed peel

12 dried apricot halves

16 oz canned pineapple pieces
(in natural juice)

$2\frac{2}{3}$ cups dark grape juice
(no added sugar)

1 tablespoon white rice flour

2 tablespoons red wine

1. Place fruits and grape juice into a medium-sized bowl.

2. Cover and allow to stand overnight.

3. The next day, pour into a medium-sized saucepan and simmer for 30 minutes or until fruit is soft.

OR The next day, pour into a microwave-safe bowl and cover with vented plastic wrap. Microwave on high for 10 minutes and stir. Microwave on medium-high (uncovered) for another 10 minutes or until fruit is soft.

4. Place rice flour into a small bowl. Blend with red wine. Stir into fruits.

5. Cook over a low heat, stirring continuously until mixture thickens.

OR Microwave on high for 1 minute and stir. Continue to microwave on high, stirring at 1 minute intervals until mixture boils and thickens.

FRUIT PLATTER WITH BERRY SAUCE

This is a delicious dessert. It is easy to prepare and is very attractive.

PREPARATION TIME: 20 minutes (to allow time to prepare fruit)
COOKING TIME: 5 minutes (3 minutes in microwave)
YIELD: 6 servings

16 oz canned raspberries, boysenberries,
or strawberries in light syrup

2 tablespoons maize corn flour

1 tablespoon sugar, as desired

2 tablespoons red wine

A selection of fruit, which may include apple,
banana, grapes, kiwifruit, pineapple,
strawberries, and so on

Lemon juice

Mint (for garnish)

1. Blend berries in an electric blender or food processor or rub through a sieve or food mill.

2. Place corn flour into a small saucepan. Stir in a little of the berry pulp and mix well. Gradually stir in remainder of the berry pulp. Cook over a low heat, stirring continuously until sauce boils and thickens.

OR Place corn flour into a small microwave-safe bowl. Stir in a little of the berry pulp and mix well. Gradually stir in remainder of the berry pulp. Microwave on high for 40 seconds and stir. Continue to microwave on high, stirring at 40 second intervals, until sauce thickens.

3. Stir sugar and red wine into sauce.

4. Allow sauce to cool.

5. Prepare fruit. Peel as necessary and cut into small pieces or slices as desired. Coat apple and banana slices with lemon juice to prevent surface browning.

6. Divide berry sauce evenly into 6 small serving bowls. Place each bowl on a flat serving plate.

7. Arrange a selection of fruits attractively on each plate and garnish with mint.

GOLDEN SYRUP DUMPLINGS

Dumplings are a very acceptable dessert in winter. They usually take a long time to cook when conventional methods are used. Cooking this recipe in the microwave oven allows the dessert to be prepared and cooked in less than 20 minutes. Dumplings are best served immediately.

PREPARATION TIME: 15 minutes • COOKING TIME: 4 minutes in microwave
YIELD: 4–6 servings

Dumplings

1⅔ cups Orgran gluten-free self-raising flour

2 tablespoons butter or salt-reduced monounsaturated margarine

⅓ cup golden syrup (such as Lyle's)

½ cup milk

Sauce

2 tablespoons butter or salt-reduced monounsaturated margarine

⅔ cup brown sugar

⅔ cup golden syrup

2 cups boiling water

2 teaspoons finely grated lemon rind

1. To make the dumplings, sift flour into a medium-sized mixing bowl. Rub butter into flour using the tips of the fingers. This process can be done using an electric food processor. Combine golden syrup and milk. Microwave on high for 40 seconds. Stir well. Make a well in the center of the dry ingredients. Pour in liquid. Stir until ingredients are well combined. Mixture should be moist and sticky.

2. To make the sauce, place all the sauce ingredients into a large microwave-safe bowl. Stir well. Microwave on high for 3 minutes. Stir and microwave for 1 minute.

3. Dust hands with gluten-free flour and roll dumpling mixture into walnut-sized balls and place into hot sauce.

4. Cover with plastic wrap. (Punch a steam outlet in the plastic wrap.)

5. Microwave on high for 4 minutes or until dumplings are well risen and firm.

LEMON MERINGUE PIE

Serve this dessert with cream, gluten-free ice cream,
or custard (see recipe page 129), as desired.

PREPARATION TIME: 30 minutes • COOKING TIME: 15 minutes for pastry case,
and 10 minutes to brown meringue

YIELD: 6 servings

Pastry

½ cup butter or salt-reduced monounsaturated margarine

3 oz sugar

½ teaspoon vanilla extract

1 egg, lightly beaten

2⅔ cups white rice flour

3 cups gluten-free, plain, all-purpose flour

½ teaspoon gluten-free baking powder

1 oz maize corn flour

1 oz gluten-free custard powder

Filling

4 tablespoons gluten-free corn flour

2 tablespoons gluten-free, plain, all-purpose flour

1⅓ cups water

½ cup sugar

1⅓ cups milk

Finely grated rind of 1 lemon

2 tablespoons butter or salt-reduced monounsaturated margarine

3 egg yolks, lightly beaten (retain whites for meringue topping)

⅔ cup lemon juice

Meringue

3 egg whites

6 tablespoons superfine sugar

Pastry

1. Preheat oven to 375°F.

2. Prepare a 9-inch pie plate by spraying with cooking spray.

3. Cream butter, sugar, and vanilla.

4. Gradually add egg to creamed mixture, beating well after each addition.

5. Sift rice flour, gluten-free flour, baking powder, corn flour, and custard powder and mix well. Mixture should be a firm consistency.

6. Turn out onto a lightly floured (gluten-free) board and knead lightly. Roll out to $\frac{1}{4}$-inch thickness.

7. Cut a circle of pastry that is 1 inch larger than pie plate. Carefully line prepared pie plate with pastry. Prick base with a fork. Moisten edge of pastry with a brush dipped in water. Roll out a $\frac{1}{2}$-inch strip of pastry to fit around edge of pie shell. (A double thickness of pastry is needed around the edge to prevent burning during cooking.)

8. Place into a moderately hot oven and bake for approximately 15 minutes or until pale golden brown.

9. While pastry case is cooking, prepare lemon filling and meringue.

10. When pastry is cooked, remove from oven and allow to cool for 5 minutes.

Filling

1. Sift corn flour and gluten-free flour into a small bowl. Blend with a little of the water. Gradually stir in remainder of water. Stir in sugar, milk, and lemon rind.

2. Pour lemon mixture into a medium-sized saucepan. Add butter. Cook over a gentle heat, stirring constantly until mixture boils and thickens. Boil for 1 minute, stirring constantly to cook the flour in the mixture.

OR Pour lemon mixture into a medium-sized microwave-safe bowl. Microwave on high for 1 minute and stir. Continue to microwave on high, stirring at 1 minute intervals until mixture boils and thickens.

3. Remove from heat. Stir in egg yolks and lemon juice and mix well.

4. Cool slightly before pouring into cooked pastry case.

5. Cover with meringue.

Meringue

1. Increase oven temperature to 400°F.

2. Place egg whites into a large, clean, dry bowl. Beat until whites are stiff.

3. Gradually add sugar and beat well until all the sugar is dissolved. Pile onto lemon filling in pastry case.

4. Place into a moderately oven and bake for approximately 10 minutes or until meringue is set and tips are golden brown. Remove from oven and serve hot or cold as desired.

MELON WITH CREAM CHEESE

This recipe can be made the day before it is required.

PREPARATION TIME: 10 minutes (+ 1 hour or more to set)
YIELD: 6–8 servings, depending on size of melon

1 melon of your choice (either cantaloupe
or honeydew melon)
3 tablespoons cold water
2 teaspoons gelatin
8 oz package light cream cheese
2 tablespoons of finely chopped ginger,
toasted almond flakes, coconut flakes,
or honey, as desired

1. Remove a ½-inch slice from the top of the melon and scoop out seeds.

2. Pour cold water into a small microwave-safe bowl. Sprinkle gelatin over water. Allow to stand for 2 minutes.

3. Microwave gelatin mixture on high for 40 seconds or until just coming to a boil. Take care not to boil mixture over.

4. Place cream cheese into a small microwave-safe bowl. Cover with paper towel and microwave for approximately 40 seconds to soften cream cheese.

5. Pour dissolved gelatin into cream cheese and stir well.

6. Add ginger (or flavor of your choice) to cream cheese. Mix well.

7. Spoon cream cheese mixture into cavity of melon, supporting melon in a round bowl so that it sits upright.

8. Refrigerate for a few hours or until required.

RHUBARB AND STRAWBERRY CRUMBLE

Serve hot or cold as desired with custard (see recipe page 129)
or gluten-free ice cream.

PREPARATION TIME: 30 minutes (allows time to cook rhubarb) •
COOKING TIME: 35 minutes (4 minutes in microwave)
YIELD: 6 servings

$5\frac{3}{4}$ cups cooked rhubarb

2 cups diced strawberries

$\frac{2}{3}$ cup brown sugar, as desired

2 tablespoons gluten-free corn flour

$\frac{1}{3}$ cup butter or salt-reduced
monounsaturated margarine

$\frac{1}{3}$ cup sugar

$\frac{2}{3}$ cup gluten-free, plain, all-purpose flour

$\frac{1}{4}$ teaspoon gluten-free baking powder

1 cup flaked almonds

1. Preheat oven to 350°F.

2. Prepare a medium-sized baking dish by spraying with cooking spray.

3. Place cooked rhubarb into prepared dish. Stir in strawberries. Mix brown sugar and corn flour together. Stir in rhubarb and strawberries.

4. In a medium-sized bowl combine butter, sugar, flour, baking powder, and almonds. Sprinkle over fruit in dish.

5. Place into a moderate oven. Bake for approximately 35 minutes or until golden brown on top.

OR Microwave on high for 4 minutes or until cooked when tested.

6. When cooked, remove from oven.

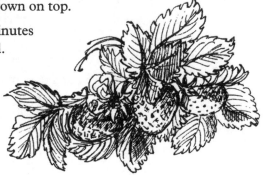

STICKY DATE PUDDING WITH BUTTERSCOTCH SAUCE

PREPARATION TIME: **15 minutes** • COOKING TIME: **40 minutes**
YIELD: **6–8 servings**

Pudding

$2\frac{1}{3}$ cups warm water

$2\frac{2}{3}$ cups finely chopped dates

$1\frac{1}{2}$ teaspoons baking soda

1 teaspoon grated fresh ginger

6 tablespoons butter or salt-reduced
monounsaturated margarine

$1\frac{1}{3}$ cups brown sugar

$\frac{1}{2}$ teaspoon vanilla extract

3 eggs

2 cups gluten-free self-raising flour

$\frac{1}{4}$ teaspoon ground cloves

$\frac{1}{2}$ teaspoon mixed spice

$\frac{1}{4}$ teaspoon nutmeg

$\frac{1}{4}$ teaspoon ground cinnamon

Butterscotch Sauce

$\frac{2}{3}$ cup butter or salt-reduced
monounsaturated margarine

$1\frac{1}{3}$ cups dark brown sugar

$\frac{1}{2}$ cup golden syrup (such as Lyle's)

1 cup light cream

1. Preheat oven to 350°F.

2. Prepare a 12- x 8-inch baking dish by spraying with cooking spray.

3. Pour water into a small saucepan. Add dates and bring to a boil. Remove from heat. Stir in baking soda and ginger. Allow to stand for 5 minutes.

4. Cream butter, sugar, and vanilla. Add eggs one at a time, beating well after each addition.

5. Sift flour and spices. Fold into creamed mixture.

6. Stir in date mixture and pour into prepared dish.

7. Bake for approximately 40 minutes or until cooked when tested.

8. When cooked, remove from oven and leave in dish to cool.

9. Serve pudding with butterscotch sauce. To make the sauce, place all the ingredients into a small saucepan and stir over a low heat. Increase heat and simmer uncovered for approximately 3 minutes or until thickened slightly.

OR Place all the ingredients into a small microwave-safe bowl. Microwave on high for 1 minute and stir. Continue to microwave for 2 minute intervals until sauce thickens slightly.

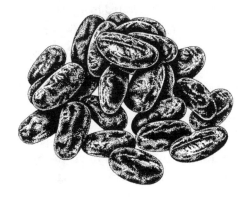

TREACLE TART

This pie has a delicious flavor. Serve warm or cold with custard (see recipe page 129) or gluten-free ice cream.

PREPARATION TIME: 20 minutes • COOKING TIME: 35 minutes
YIELD: 6 servings

Filling

$^2/_3$ cup treacle (such as Lyle's treacle,
or substitute Lyle's golden syrup)

2 teaspoons finely grated lemon rind

1$^2/_3$ cups gluten-free bread crumbs

Pastry

1 cup white rice flour

1$^1/_3$ cups gluten-free, plain, all-purpose flour

1 teaspoon gluten-free baking powder

6 tablespoons salt-reduced
monounsaturated margarine

$^2/_3$ cup finely granulated white sugar

3$^1/_2$ fl oz low-fat milk, approximately

Filling

1. Place all the ingredients into a small saucepan. Cook over a low heat, stirring continuously to combine ingredients. Remove from heat.

OR Place all the ingredients into a small microwave-safe bowl. Microwave on high for 1 minute. Stir and microwave again on high for 1 minute.

2. Set filling aside while preparing pastry.

Pastry

1. Preheat oven to 350°F.

2. Prepare a 9-inch pie dish by spraying with cooking spray.

3. Sift rice flour, gluten-free plain flour, and baking powder into a medium-sized mixing bowl.

4. Rub margarine into dry ingredients until mixture resembles fine bread crumbs. This process may be done by hand or with the aid of an electric food processor.

5. Stir in sugar and sufficient milk to mix to a firm dough.

6. Turn dough out onto a lightly floured (gluten-free) board and knead lightly.

7. Gently roll out pastry to approximately $\frac{1}{4}$-inch thickness.

8. Carefully line base of prepared pie dish with pastry, reserving enough pastry to decorate top of pie.

9. Pour treacle filling onto prepared pie base.

10. Cut remaining pastry into $\frac{1}{2}$-inch-wide strips and decorate top of pie.

11. Place pie into oven and bake for approximately 35 minutes or until firm to touch and lightly golden brown.

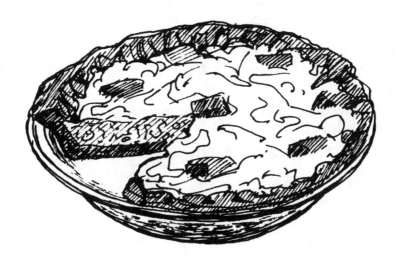

TROPICAL TRIFLE

This trifle is set in layers and has great appeal for serving.
This has been a family favorite with my friend Bryan. Serve hot or
cold with whipped cream or gluten-free ice cream, as desired.

PREPARATION TIME: 60 minutes (allowing time for Jell-O to set and to make custard; pineapple cake can be made ahead of time)

YIELD: 8 servings

1 pineapple cake (see recipe on page 180)
$\frac{1}{3}$ cup cream sherry
14 oz canned pineapple pieces
1 package pineapple Jell-O
1 package orange Jell-O
1 quantity custard (see recipe on page 129)

1. Cut pineapple cake into 1-inch cubes and place into the base of a 9-inch round serving plate.

2. Pour sherry over cake. Allow to soak into cake while preparing Jell-O.

3. Strain juice from pineapple pieces and reserve pieces and juice.

4. Make up pineapple Jell-O according to package instructions. Use juice from pineapple and make up to required liquid with water. Pour over cake. Allow to set.

5. Make up orange Jell-O according to package instructions. Pour over pineapple Jell-O. Allow to set.

6. Pour custard onto set Jell-O. Refrigerate until required.

7. Arrange pineapple pieces on custard for serving.

8. Cut into slices for serving.

9.

Holiday Fare

Almond Loaf, 144
Cherry Chutney, 146
Chocolates, 147
Christmas Pudding, 148
Festival Cake, 150
Fruit Mince Pies, 151
Fruitcake, 154
Shortbread, 156

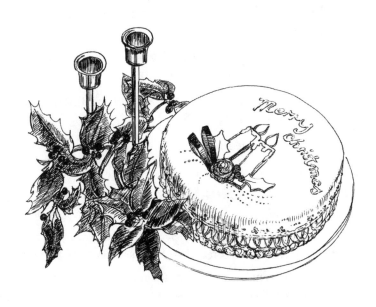

ALMOND LOAF

*This is a bread that is traditionally served in Australia at Christmas time.
It will remain crisp when stored in an airtight container. Other nuts
and/or dried fruits can be substituted for almonds. This bread is baked,
allowed to cool, and then thinly sliced and dried out in a very slow oven.
It will cut best if it is partly frozen before thinly slicing.*

PREPARATION TIME: 15 minutes • COOKING TIME: 40 minutes
(allow approximately 1$\frac{1}{2}$ hours for drying time)
YIELD: Approximately 24 slices, depending on the thickness
of each slice (the slices are best if they are cut thinly)

3 egg whites

Pinch salt

$\frac{2}{3}$ cup finely granulated white sugar

1$\frac{1}{3}$ cup gluten-free, plain, all-purpose flour

11 oz almonds*

$\frac{1}{4}$ teaspoon vanilla extract**

1. Preheat oven to 300°F.

2. Prepare a 10- x 3$\frac{1}{4}$-inch loaf pan by spraying with cooking spray. Line
   base of pan with baking paper.

3. Place egg whites into a large, clean, dry bowl. Add a pinch of salt and
   beat until egg whites hold stiff peaks.

4. Gradually add sugar, beating well after each addition, until all the
   sugar is thoroughly dissolved.

5. Gently fold in gluten-free flour.

6. Gently stir in almonds and vanilla.

7. Spread into prepared pan. Smooth surface with a spatula dipped in
   water.

---

 * Use almonds with brown skins on as this gives the best appearance when sliced.

** It is best to use pure vanilla extract and not imitation vanilla for this recipe. If
   you use too much vanilla in the mixture, it will give a slight discoloration to the
   finished product.

8. Place into a moderately slow oven and bake for approximately 40 minutes or until firm to touch and cooked when tested.

9. Allow to cool in pan for 15 minutes. Turn out of pan and remove baking paper.

10. Wrap in plastic wrap and allow to completely cool. Place into freezer for approximately 1 hour. Cut into $1/4$-inch slices.

11. Prepare two large, flat baking trays by lightly spraying with cooking spray. Place slices onto prepared tray. DO NOT overlap slices. Place into a very slow oven 225°F for approximately 40 minutes. Turn slices over and continue to dry out for approximately 40 minutes longer. Take care not to brown slices as they should be white in color when the drying process is completed.

12. Remove from oven and allow to cool. When cold, remove from trays and store in an airtight container.

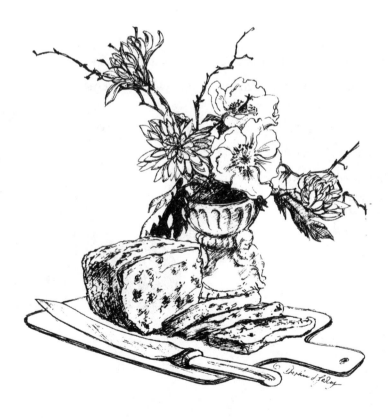

CHERRY CHUTNEY

Cherry chutney is a favorite in our family when served with ham at Christmas. We choose to serve it with turkey instead of the traditional cranberry sauce.

PREPARATION TIME: 30 minutes (to allow time to remove pits from cherries) • COOKING TIME: 20 minutes
YIELD: 6 x 10 fl oz jars

2 lbs cherries

1 large red onion, peeled and finely diced

$\frac{1}{2}$ teaspoon cinnamon

2 cups sugar

$\frac{1}{3}$ cup balsamic vinegar

Juice of 1 lemon

$\frac{1}{2}$ cup olive oil

$\frac{2}{3}$ cup port

1. Remove pits from cherries. Cut cherries in half.

2. Place cherries, onion, cinnamon, sugar, vinegar, lemon juice, and oil into a large saucepan.

3. Cook over a gentle heat until mixture thickens.

4. Stir in port. Cook for 1 minute.

5. When cooked, bottle in warm sterilized jars and seal. Store in the refrigerator.

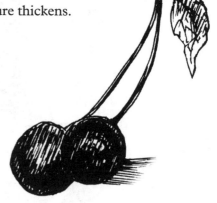

CHOCOLATES

This recipe is a "sometimes" food for special occasions. It is designed for those who wish to make their own gluten-free chocolates. Carob buttons may be used instead of chocolate if desired.

PREPARATION TIME: 20 minutes • COOKING TIME: 5 minutes
YIELD: Approximately 40 chocolates

1 egg yolk

$^2/_3$ cup pure icing sugar (sifted)

4 tablespoons soft unsalted butter or
salt-reduced monounsaturated margarine

1 teaspoon vanilla extract

1 tablespoon brandy

6 oz good-quality dark compounded
cooking chocolate

1. Prepare a large, flat tray by covering with plastic wrap or baking paper.

2. Place egg yolk, icing sugar, butter, vanilla, and brandy into the small bowl of an electric food mixer. Mix ingredients well together.

3. Place chocolate into the top of a double saucepan. Melt chocolate over a low heat.

OR Place chocolate into a microwave-safe bowl. Microwave on medium-high for 1 minute and stir. Continue to microwave on medium-high, stirring at 30 second intervals, until chocolate is melted.

4. Pour melted chocolate into ingredients in bowl, beating all the time. Mix thoroughly.

5. Allow mixture to firm a little if necessary before using.

6. Spoon mixture into a piping bag with a large star nozzle.

7. Pipe stars onto prepared tray.

8. Refrigerate until required.

CHRISTMAS PUDDING

This is a rich, moist Christmas pudding designed for those who cannot tolerate gluten in their diet. The recipe uses no eggs. The flavor in this pudding will develop best if it is cooked at least 1 week before serving. Serve with custard (see recipe page 129).

PREPARATION TIME: 30 minutes • COOKING TIME: 3 hours
YIELD: 8 servings

6 tablespoons butter or salt reduced
monounsaturated margarine

4 oz brown sugar

$\frac{1}{2}$ teaspoon vanilla extract

6 oz currants

6 oz finely chopped golden raisins (sultanas)

6 oz finely chopped raisins

2 oz (60 g) mixed peel

2 large green cooking apples,
peeled and grated

Finely grated rind of 1 orange

3 oz gluten-free bread crumbs

$\frac{1}{2}$ cup rum

2 tablespoons maize corn flour

$1\frac{1}{3}$ cup gluten-free, plain, all-purpose flour

1 teaspoon Ener-G Egg Replacer or
Orgran No Egg

$\frac{1}{4}$ teaspoon baking soda

1 teaspoon cinnamon

$\frac{1}{2}$ teaspoon nutmeg

$\frac{2}{3}$ cup polenta

2 tablespoons rice bran

1. Prepare a large bowl by spraying with cooking spray.

2. Cut a large enough circle of baking paper to cover top and part of side of bowl. Cut out a circle of foil the same size as baking paper.

3. Pour a small quantity of water into a large saucepan and boil.

4. Cream margarine, sugar, and vanilla.

5. Stir dried fruits, mixed peel, grated apple, orange rind, bread crumbs, and rum into creamed mixture.

6. Sift corn flour, gluten-free flour, egg substitute, baking soda, and spices into a small bowl. Stir in polenta and rice bran. Add to fruit mixture and mix well.

7. Place mixture into prepared bowl.

8. Cover bowl with baking paper and secure. Cover with foil and secure.

9. Carefully lower bowl into boiling water in saucepan. If necessary, add more boiling water so that water reaches halfway up side of bowl. Place lid on saucepan.

10. Boil continuously for 3 hours. If necessary, add more boiling water during cooking.

11. Remove pudding from boiling water and leave in basin to cool.

12. When cold, wrap securely in foil and store in refrigerator until required.

13. On the day you are serving, re-steam for 1 hour if required hot. Turn out onto a serving plate and serve as desired.

OR On the day you are serving, slices of pudding may be warmed in the microwave oven. Allow approximately 1 minute on high for each cold slice. Serve as desired.

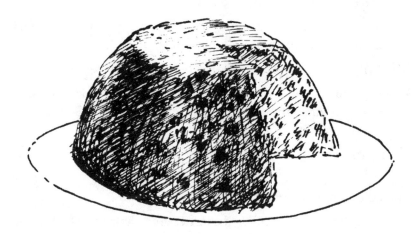

Festival Cake

This is a delicious cake made from a selection of dried and candied fruits. It can be made up to three months before needed and stored in the refrigerator.

PREPARATION TIME: 17 minutes • COOKING TIME: 1 hour

4 oz candied pineapple

4 oz candied apricot

8 oz bag pitted dates

8 oz mixed-colored candied cherries

4 oz whole blanched almonds

8 oz Brazil nuts

2 eggs

$^{2}/_{3}$ cup brown sugar

6 tablespoons soft butter or salt-reduced
monounsaturated margarine

1 tablespoon cherry brandy

$^{1}/_{2}$ teaspoon vanilla extract

$^{1}/_{2}$ cup gluten-free, plain, all-purpose flour

$^{1}/_{2}$ cup gluten-free self-raising flour

2 oz red candied cherries, extra

2 oz whole blanched almonds, extra

1. Preheat oven to 325°F.

2. Prepare two 10- x 3-inch loaf pans by spraying with cooking spray. Line base of pans with baking paper.

3. Chop pineapple and apricot into small pieces approximately 1 inch in size. Leave dates, cherries, and nuts whole.

4. Mix fruit and nuts together.

5. In a separate clean, dry bowl, beat eggs until thick and creamy. Add sugar to mixture, mixing well after each addition. Stir in butter, brandy, and vanilla.

6. Sift flours into a small bowl. Stir in fruits. Stir into egg mixture, mixing well.

7. Spread mixture into prepared pans.

8. Decorate each with red candied cherries and whole blanched almonds.

9. Place into a moderate oven and bake for approximately 1 hour or until cake is cooked when tested.

10. When cooked, remove from oven and allow to cool in pan for 10 minutes before turning out onto a fine wire rack to cool.

11. Seal with plastic wrap while still warm. This allows cake to remain moist. Allow to cool completely before placing into an airtight container. Refrigerate until required.

FRUIT MINCE PIES

These fruit mince mini pies or tarts are delicious Christmas treats. As a variation, fruit mince slice can be made by using half the pastry to line a cake pan. Fruit mince can be spread over pastry and remaining pastry rolled out and placed on top.

PREPARATION TIME: 30 minutes (Fruit mince can be made ahead of time and stored in an airtight container in the refrigerator until required) • COOKING TIME: 13 minutes
YIELD: Approximately 24 pies

Fruit Mince

1 cooking apple, peeled and grated

15 oz can crushed pineapple in natural juice

$1\frac{1}{3}$ cup natural golden raisins (sultanas)

$1\frac{1}{3}$ cup chopped natural raisins

$\frac{2}{3}$ cup currants

2 oz candied cherries, cut in half

1 tablespoon brown sugar

1 tablespoon butter or salt-reduced monounsaturated margarine

Finely grated rind 1 lemon

1 teaspoon ground cinnamon

$\frac{1}{2}$ teaspoon ground nutmeg

1 tablespoon gluten-free corn flour

$\frac{1}{3}$ cup brandy

Pastry for Pies

$\frac{1}{2}$ cup butter or salt-reduced
monounsaturated margarine

$\frac{2}{3}$ cup finely granulated white sugar

$\frac{1}{2}$ teaspoon vanilla extract

1 egg, lightly beaten

3 oz white rice flour

3 oz brown rice flour

3 oz gluten-free bread mix

$\frac{1}{2}$ teaspoon gluten-free
baking powder

1 oz gluten-free corn flour

1 oz gluten-free custard powder

Pure icing sugar, to sprinkle on top
of cooked pies

Fruit Mince

1. Place all the ingredients except the corn flour and brandy into a medium-sized saucepan. Stir over a gentle heat until all the ingredients are well combined and mixture boils. Cook over a gentle heat, stirring occasionally to prevent mixture from sticking.

OR Place all the ingredients except the corn flour and brandy into a medium-sized microwave-safe bowl. Microwave on high for 2 minutes and stir. Microwave on medium-high stirring at 1 minute intervals until mixture is softened and well combined.

2. Place corn flour into a small bowl. Blend with brandy. Mix into hot fruit, stirring continuously.

3. Return to heat and cook until mixture comes to a boil, stirring continuously.

OR Microwave on high for 1 minute and stir. Microwave on medium for 1 minute.

4. Allow to cool and store in a covered container in the refrigerator until required as filling.

Pastry for Pies

1. Preheat oven to 400°F.

2. Individual foil trays are best for making these mini pies or tarts.

3. Cream butter, sugar, and vanilla.

4. Gradually add egg to creamed mixture, beating well after each addition.

5. Sift rice flours, gluten-free bread mix, baking powder, corn flour, and custard powder into creamed mixture and mix well. Dough should be a firm consistency.

6. Turn pastry out onto a lightly floured (gluten-free) board and knead lightly. Divide pastry in half. Roll half the pastry to approximately $1/4$-inch thickness.

7. Using a $2^1/_2$-inch fluted cutter dipped in gluten-free flour, cut out rounds of pastry.

8. Carefully lift into individual foil trays and gently press pastry into each foil tray.

9. Place pie shells onto a flat oven tray and place 1 tablespoon fruit mince into each pie shell.

10. Roll out remaining pastry to approximately $1/4$-inch thickness. Using a $1^1/_4$-inch fluted cutter, cut out small rounds of pastry. Place a top onto each pie.

11. Place into a moderately hot oven and bake for 5 minutes. Reduce heat to 350°F and bake for another 8 minutes or until pastry is lightly golden brown.

12. When cooked, remove from oven and leave in foil trays to cool. Store in a covered container in the refrigerator.

13. Just before serving, lightly dust with pure icing sugar.

FRUITCAKE

Gluten-free fruitcakes are a very pleasant addition to the holiday fare.
For best results, soak the fruit in gin overnight or for up to one week.
Cake will develop in flavor if made two to four weeks before it is required.
When the cake is cooked, it is best wrapped in several thicknesses
of newspaper and left until it cools completely. It can be stored
in this wrapping until it is required.

PREPARATION TIME: **30 minutes** • COOKING TIME: **3 hours**

8 oz finely chopped raisins

8 oz natural golden raisins
(sultanas)

8 oz currants

4 oz mixed peel

1 cup gin

4 oz blanched almonds

Finely grated rind of 1 orange

Finely grated rind of 1 lemon

2 tablespoons marmalade

1 cup butter or salt-reduced
monounsaturated margarine

8 oz brown sugar

1 tablespoon treacle
(such as Lyle's treacle)

1 teaspoon vanilla extract

3 eggs

10 oz gluten-free, plain, all-purpose flour

2 oz gluten-free self-raising flour

$\frac{1}{2}$ teaspoon baking soda

$\frac{1}{2}$ teaspoon each of cinnamon,
grated nutmeg, ground ginger

1 teaspoon mixed spice

2 tablespoons gin extra
(to pour over cake after it is cooked)

1. Preheat oven to 300°F.

2. Prepare a 9-inch round cake pan by spraying with cooking spray. Line base and sides of pan with baking paper.

3. Cut out three layers of brown paper to wrap around outside and bottom of pan. Secure brown paper to pan with string. You will also need a sheet of brown paper to cover top of cake during cooking.

4. Place fruits, peel, gin, almonds, rinds, and marmalade into a large mixing bowl and mix well.

5. Cream margarine, sugar, treacle, and vanilla.

6. Add eggs one at a time, beating well after each addition.

7. Sift flours, baking soda, and spices into a small bowl.

8. Add fruit mixture and sifted dry ingredients alternately to creamed mixture, mixing well after each addition.

9. Spread mixture into prepared pan. Bump pan a few times to remove air bubbles. Cover with brown paper.

10. Place cake into oven and bake for 30 minutes.

11. Reduce heat to 250°F and bake for another 2 hours. Remove brown paper from top of cake and bake for another 30 minutes or until cooked when tested.

12. When cooked, remove from oven. Slowly pour extra 2 tablespoons gin over top of cake in pan.

13. Place a sheet of greaseproof or brown paper on top of cake in pan and wrap in several thicknesses of newspaper.

14. Allow to cool overnight before unwrapping.

SHORTBREAD

*The holidays are a time for enjoyment of food. There is no reason
why you cannot enjoy your favorite treats on a gluten-free diet.
One tablespoon of whiskey can be added with the honey if desired.*

PREPARATION TIME: 20 minutes • COOKING TIME: 45 minutes
YIELD: Approximately 12 pieces depending on size

$1\frac{1}{2}$ cups butter or
monounsaturated margarine

6 oz pure icing sugar

$\frac{1}{2}$ teaspoon vanilla extract

2 tablespoons honey

$3\frac{1}{2}$ oz white rice flour

13 oz gluten-free, plain,
all-purpose flour

1. Preheat oven to 325°F.

2. Prepare a $9\frac{1}{2}$- x 8- x $\frac{1}{2}$-inch flat oven tray by spraying with cooking spray.

3. Cream margarine, icing sugar, vanilla, and honey.

4. Add rice flour and gluten-free flour to creamed mixture and mix well.

5. Press mixture into prepared tray.

6. Decorate with a pattern as desired.

7. Place shortbread into oven and bake for approximately 45 minutes or until very pale golden brown.

8. When cooked, remove from oven and leave in tray for 2 minutes.

9. Cut into squares and leave in tray to cool.

10. When cold, carefully remove from tray and store in an airtight container.

10.

Goodies
to Bake

Cookies

Anzac Cookies, 158

Chocolate Brownies, 160

Coffee Cream Cookies, 161

Custard Cookies, 163

Edna's Kisses, 164

Honey Cookies, 165

Walnut-Cinnamon Cookies,
166

Cakes

Apple Slice, 169

Apple and Date Slice, 170

Apple Tea Cake, 171

Butter Cake, 172

Carrot Cake, 173

Chocolate-Almond Cake,
174

Chocolate-Banana Cake, 175

Chocolate Mud Cake, 176

Date Fudge Slice, 177

Ginger Cake, 178

Pecan Cake, 179

Pineapple Cake, 180

Plain Cake (with variations),
181

Poppy Seed Cake, 182

Silver Cake, 183

Spicy Coffee Cake, 184

Zucchini Cake, 185

COOKIES

Following are some delicious cookie recipes, and one for brownies—
all gluten-free.

ANZAC COOKIES

*Anzac cookies originated during World War I when the women
in Australia decided to send some cooking to the Anzacs, the men of
the Australia and New Zealand Army Corps. The original ingredients
were chosen for their excellent keeping qualities, as they had to
survive a long sea voyage of about two months to get to
the soldiers on the barren slopes of Gallipoli.*

*Oat is a very nutritious cereal, containing the most protein of
any cereal. The original recipe is supposed to be based on an old
Scottish recipe for oatmeal cookies. Coconut and golden syrup were
added to the original recipe of rolled oats, butter, sugar, and flour.
The cookies did not have eggs as these were in short supply during
war years. After the war, fundraising activities were set up with
Anzac cookie drives to raise money for injured war veterans.
The cookies became popular again during World War II.*

*The original Anzac cookie recipe is adapted here
to make a gluten-free product.*

PREPARATION TIME: 15 minutes • COOKING TIME: 15 minutes
YIELD: Approximately 24 cookies

$1\frac{1}{3}$ cups white rice flour

$1\frac{1}{3}$ cups rolled rice flakes

2 tablespoons rice bran

$\frac{2}{3}$ cup sugar

1 cup desiccated coconut

$\frac{1}{2}$ cup butter or salt-reduced
monounsaturated margarine

2 tablespoons golden syrup (such as Lyle's)

$\frac{1}{3}$ teaspoon vanilla extract

$\frac{1}{2}$ teaspoon baking soda

1 tablespoon boiling water

1. Preheat oven to 325°F.

2. Prepare two flat oven trays by spraying with cooking spray.

3. Sift rice flour into a large mixing bowl. Place rolled rice, rice bran, sugar, and coconut into bowl.

4. Place butter into a small saucepan and melt over a gentle heat. Stir in golden syrup and vanilla.

OR Place butter into a small microwave-safe bowl. Cover and microwave on high for 40 seconds or until butter is melted. Stir in golden syrup and vanilla.

5. Mix baking soda with boiling water and add to warmed liquid. Stir liquid into dry ingredients and mix well. Mixture should be a moist consistency.

6. Lightly dust hands with gluten-free flour and roll portions of mixture into walnut-sized balls and place onto prepared trays. Use a fork dipped in gluten-free flour to press flat.

7. Place into a moderately slow oven and bake for approximately 15 minutes or until golden brown.

8. When cooked, remove from oven and leave on trays for 2 minutes. Loosen cookies and leave on trays to cool.

9. When cold, store in an airtight container.

CHOCOLATE BROWNIES

These brownies are a favorite with my friend Diane.

PREPARATION TIME: 15 minutes • COOKING TIME: 35 minutes
YIELD: 16 brownies

5 oz dark chocolate

$^2/_3$ cup butter or salt-reduced
monounsaturated margarine

2 medium eggs

6 oz finely granulated white sugar

$3^1/_2$ oz gluten-free, plain, all-purpose flour

$3^1/_2$ oz chopped walnuts

1. Preheat oven to 350°F.

2. Prepare an 8-inch square cake pan by spraying with cooking spray. Line pan with baking paper.

3. Place chocolate and butter into a small heatproof bowl. Stir over hot water, until chocolate is melted.

4. Place eggs and sugar into a medium-sized bowl. Beat until slightly thickened. Stir in melted chocolate mixture.

5. Stir in flour and walnuts.

6. Pour mixture into prepared pan.

7. Place into a moderate oven and bake for approximately 35 minutes or until set in the center.

8. When cooked, remove from oven and leave to cool in the pan for 5–10 minutes.

9. Carefully remove from pan and turn out onto a wire rack to cool completely.

10. When cold, cut into squares.

COFFEE CREAM COOKIES

While I was creating new recipes for this book, I attended training sessions for a church group working to minister to relatives with loved ones in jail. Out of a group of thirty women in the training team, five required a gluten-free diet. I used to take different gluten-free foods for morning tea. This recipe was voted the nicest cookie of all the cookies sampled by the group. It originated as a recipe my mother used to make in the 1950s. It has since then been a favorite in our home and now, of course, it is a gluten-free favorite.

PREPARATION TIME: 30 minutes • COOKING TIME: 15 minutes
YIELD: Approximately 12 filled cookies

Cookies

6 tablespoons butter or salt-reduced
monounsaturated margarine

3 oz finely granulated white sugar

$\frac{1}{2}$ teaspoon vanilla extract

1 egg, lightly beaten

1$\frac{1}{3}$ cups gluten-free self-raising flour

$\frac{1}{3}$ cup gluten-free, plain, all-purpose flour

$\frac{1}{3}$ cup gluten-free corn flour

2 teaspoons instant coffee powder

Coffee Cream

2 tablespoons butter or salt-reduced
monounsaturated margarine

$\frac{1}{2}$ teaspoon instant coffee powder

3 oz pure icing sugar, sifted

Hot water, to mix

1. Preheat oven to 350°F.

2. Prepare two flat oven trays by spraying with cooking spray.

3. Cream butter, sugar, and vanilla. Gradually add egg to creamed mixture, beating well after each addition.

4. Sift flours and corn flour into a small bowl. Stir in coffee powder. Mix into creamed mixture.

5. Lightly dust hands with gluten-free flour and roll portions of mixture into walnut-sized balls and place onto prepared trays. Use a fork dipped in gluten-free flour to press flat.

6. Place into a moderate oven and bake for approximately 15 minutes or until golden brown.

7. When cooked, remove from oven and leave on trays for 2 minutes. Loosen cookies and leave on trays while preparing the coffee cream.

8. To make the coffee cream, place butter into a bowl. Soften butter by beating well with a wooden spoon. Add coffee powder and icing sugar and beat well. Mix to a smooth paste with a little hot water.

9. While cookies are still warm, top with coffee cream.

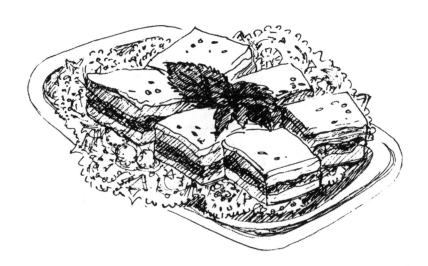

CUSTARD COOKIES

These crisp cookies are a favorite recipe in our home.

PREPARATION TIME: 15 minutes • COOKING TIME: 15 minutes
YIELD: Approximately 24 cookies

½ cup butter or salt-reduced
monounsaturated margarine

4 oz finely granulated white sugar

½ teaspoon vanilla extract

1 egg

1⅔ cups gluten-free, plain,
all-purpose flour

⅔ cup white rice flour

⅓ cup gluten-free custard powder

1 teaspoon gluten-free baking powder

1. Preheat oven to 350°F.

2. Prepare two flat oven trays by spraying with cooking spray.

3. Cream butter, sugar, and vanilla.

4. Lightly beat egg. Pour into creamed mixture and beat well.

5. Sift gluten-free flour, rice flour, custard powder, and baking powder into a small bowl.

6. Add sifted dry ingredients to creamed mixture and mix well.

7. Lightly dust hands with gluten-free powder and roll mixture into walnut-sized balls and place onto prepared trays. Gently flatten balls with a fork dipped in gluten-free flour.

8. Place cookies into oven and bake for approximately 15 minutes or until pale golden brown.

9. When cooked, remove from oven and leave on trays for 2 minutes. Loosen cookies and leave on trays to cool.

10. When cold, remove from trays and store in an airtight container.

EDNA'S KISSES

This is a very old-fashioned recipe. The result is a delicious, melt-in-the-mouth sensation that will delight your palate. A very dear lady in our church, Edna, has made the recipe for about sixty years. She says it was grandma Marion Gibson's recipe. When my friend Susan's niece Sara was diagnosed with celiac disease, Susan took the traditional recipe that has stood the test of time and made it gluten-free. These cookies are a favorite for Sara and for others who have tasted the lovely product.

The recipe is made up by weighing the eggs and measuring the ingredients according to the weight of the eggs. If you have heavier eggs you will have more gluten-free flour, butter, sugar, and corn flour, and you will of course make more cookies. I have used Orgran gluten-free, plain, all-purpose flour in this recipe.

PREPARATION TIME: 15 minutes • COOKING TIME: 12–15 minutes
YIELD: 20 cookies when joined together with jam

$\frac{1}{2}$ cup butter
4 oz finely granulated white sugar
$\frac{1}{4}$ teaspoon vanilla extract
2 eggs (2 oz each)
4 oz Orgran gluten-free, plain,
all-purpose flour
4 oz gluten-free corn flour
1 teaspoon gluten-free baking powder
Jam of your choice

1. Preheat oven to 350°F.

2. Prepare a flat baking tray by spraying with cooking spray. Line tray with baking paper.

3. Cream butter, sugar, and vanilla.

4. Beat eggs and add to creamed mixture.

5. Sift gluten-free flour, corn flour, and baking powder into a medium-sized bowl. Lightly fold into creamed mixture.

6. Drop teaspoons of mixture onto prepared tray.

7. Place into a moderate oven and bake for approximately 12–15 minutes or until cooked. Take care not to overcook, as kisses should be pale in color.

8. When cooked, remove from oven. Leave cookies on tray for 5 minutes. Remove from tray and place onto a fine wire rack to cool.

9. When cold, join the cookies with a thin layer of jam. Jam will be easier to spread if it is warmed for a few seconds in the microwave.

HONEY COOKIES

These cookies have a crisp texture with a nice honey flavor.

PREPARATION TIME: 15 minutes • COOKING TIME: 15 minutes
YIELD: Approximately 50 cookies

1 cup butter or salt-reduced monounsaturated margarine
$2/3$ cup brown sugar
$2/3$ cup honey
1 teaspoon vanilla extract
$2^2/3$ cups white rice flour
$2^2/3$ cups gluten-free, plain, all-purpose flour
2 teaspoons gluten-free baking powder

1. Preheat oven to 350°F.

2. Prepare two flat oven trays by spraying with cooking spray.

3. Cream butter, sugar, honey, and vanilla.

4. Sift rice flours, gluten-free flour, and baking powder into a small bowl.

5. Add sifted dry ingredients to creamed mixture and mix well.

6. Lightly dust hands with gluten-free flour and roll mixture into walnut-sized balls and place onto prepared trays. Gently flatten balls with a fork dipped in gluten-free flour.

7. Place cookies into oven and bake for approximately 15 minutes or until golden brown.

8. When cooked, remove from oven and leave on trays for 2 minutes. Loosen cookies and leave on trays to cool.

9. When cold, remove cookies from trays and store in an airtight container.

WALNUT-CINNAMON COOKIES

PREPARATION TIME: 15 minutes • COOKING TIME: 15 minutes
YIELD: Approximately 40 cookies

1 cup butter or salt-reduced
monounsaturated margarine

8 oz finely granulated white sugar

$\frac{1}{2}$ teaspoon vanilla extract

2 eggs, lightly beaten

4 oz walnut pieces

10 oz brown rice flour

5 oz gluten-free, plain,
all-purpose flour

1 teaspoon gluten-free
baking powder

1 teaspoon cinnamon

1. Preheat oven to 325°F.

2. Prepare two flat oven trays by spraying with cooking spray.

3. Cream butter, sugar, and vanilla.

4. Gradually add egg to creamed mixture, beating well after each addition.

5. Stir in walnuts.

6. Sift brown rice flour, gluten-free plain flour, baking powder, and cinnamon into creamed mixture and mix well. Mixture should be a firm consistency.

7. Lightly dust hands with gluten-free flour and roll portions of mixture into walnut-sized balls and place onto prepared trays. Use a fork dipped in gluten-free flour to press flat.

8. Place into a moderately slow oven and bake for approximately 15 minutes or until golden brown.

9. When cooked, remove cookies from oven and leave on trays for 2 minutes. Loosen cookies and leave on trays to cool.

10. When cold, store in an airtight container.

CAKES

Gluten is made up of many proteins, some of which are soluble and some insoluble. These proteins are divided into two parts, known as gliadin and glutenin. When gluten in wheaten flour is moistened, it forms a cohesive, elastic network due to the cross-linkages between the protein molecules. The cohesiveness of the gluten in association with a raising agent enables baked flour products to increase in size. The flour stretches when the raising agent is activated by the addition of sufficient moisture and heat, and sets on baking in its risen position.

An absence of gluten in a cake can result in the cake rising and then sinking in the middle. This may be prevented by:

1. Adding ascorbic acid. Crush and add one 25-milligram vitamin C tablet to each cake mixture.

2. Using a ring cake pan for baking cakes.

3. Substituting one of the flours in the recipe with one of the following:
   - $\frac{1}{3}$ to $\frac{2}{3}$ cup soy flour.
   - $\frac{1}{3}$ to $\frac{2}{3}$ cup gluten-free instant infant rice cereal. (Rice cereal has pre-gelling properties that help bind the baked product. Take care to read all labels before purchasing.)
   - $\frac{1}{3}$ to $\frac{2}{3}$ cup rice bran.

4. Substituting gluten-free flour in place of gluten flour.

5. Adding 1 teaspoon of a pre-gel starch such as xanthan gum.

6. Using Orgran gluten-free gluten substitute.

It is best to use nonstick cake pans when baking cakes as this will make it easier to remove soft cakes from the pan. It is necessary to grease these pans when making gluten-free cakes.

After cakes are removed from the oven, leave in pans for 10 minutes before turning out onto a fine wire rack to cool. This will allow the cake to cool slightly before it is removed from the pan and help prevent soft cakes from breaking.

If you find it difficult to cut gluten-free cakes, place them into the freezer for approximately 1 hour before slicing. You will find cake will slice more easily and will be less likely to crumble.

Flours Suitable for Gluten-Free Cakes

Arrowroot: This starch is made from the tuber of a West Indian plant.

Buckwheat flour: Buckwheat is not a cereal. It is an herbaceous plant whose seed is ground into flour.

Corn flour: Corn flour can be made from either maize or wheat. When following a gluten-free diet, use maize corn flour. Maize corn flour is produced from 100 percent corn and is therefore suitable for a gluten-free diet.

Gluten-free flour: A wide selection is now available at supermarkets and health food stores.

Lentil flour: Made from lentils.

Pea flour: Made from peas; also known as besan flour.

Potato flour: This is produced from the starch of the potato.

Rice flour: White and brown rice flours are available.

Soy flour: This is made from ground soybeans.

APPLE SLICE

Apple slice is delicious served hot or cold.

PREPARATION TIME: 20 minutes • COOKING TIME: 30 minutes

$\frac{1}{2}$ cup butter or salt-reduced monounsaturated margarine

$\frac{2}{3}$ cup superfine sugar

$\frac{1}{2}$ teaspoon vanilla extract

1 egg

1$\frac{1}{3}$ cups white rice flour

1$\frac{1}{3}$ cups gluten-free, plain, all-purpose flour

2 teaspoons gluten-free baking powder

2$\frac{2}{3}$ cups cold, cooked apple (approx. 5 large cooking apples)

1 teaspoon cinnamon

1 egg white, lightly beaten

$\frac{2}{3}$ cup almond flakes

2 teaspoons raw sugar

1. Preheat oven to 400°F.

2. Prepare a 9-inch square cake pan by spraying with cooking spray.

3. Cream margarine, sugar, and vanilla.

4. Add egg and beat well.

5. Sift rice flour, gluten-free flour, and baking powder into creamed mixture and mix to a firm dough.

6. Turn dough out onto a lightly floured (gluten-free) board and knead lightly. Divide pastry in half. Carefully roll out half the pastry to approximately $\frac{1}{4}$-inch thickness to fit base of pan.

7. Line base of prepared pan with rolled out pastry. Spread apple evenly over pastry. Sprinkle cinnamon over apple.

8. Carefully roll out remainder of pastry and cover apple.

9. Brush top of pastry with a little egg white. Sprinkle almond flakes and raw sugar evenly over pastry.

10. Place slice into oven and bake for 10 minutes. Reduce heat to 350°F and bake for another 20 minutes or until pastry is cooked.

11. When cooked, remove from oven and leave in pan to cool.

APPLE AND DATE SLICE

One of my greatest joys in life is when I go to a friend's house and they make me a gluten-free recipe. One such occasion when this happened was while I was visiting Tasmania. My friend Laurie converted a family favorite recipe to gluten-free. What a joy it was one evening when I was his house guest to be treated to lovely coffee and this delicious slice.

When Laurie made the slice he used rice flour. I make it with Orgran flour. Also, mixed fruit or any dried fruit can be substituted for dates. Half a cup of coconut can be added if desired.

PREPARATION TIME: **20 minutes** • COOKING TIME: **25 minutes**

$1\frac{1}{3}$ cups diced cooked apple

6 oz brown sugar

1 cup salt-reduced monounsaturated margarine

2 tablespoons golden syrup (such as Lyle's)

1 egg

$\frac{1}{2}$ teaspoon vanilla extract

$1\frac{1}{3}$ cups finely chopped dates

4 oz Orgran gluten-free, plain, all-purpose flour

4 oz gluten-free self-raising flour

$\frac{1}{4}$ teaspoon baking soda

1. Preheat oven to 350°F.

2. Prepare 7- x 10-inch cake tray by spraying with cooking spray.

3. Place hot apple into a mixing bowl. Mix in sugar, margarine, and golden syrup. Allow to cool slightly.

4. Lightly beat egg. Add vanilla and mix well. Add egg and vanilla to apple and mix well. Stir in dates.

5. Stir flours and baking soda into apple mixture and mix well. Spread into prepared pan.

6. Place into a moderate oven and bake for approximately 25 minutes or until cooked when tested. Leave in tray for 10 minutes before cutting into squares.

APPLE TEA CAKE

When making gluten-free baked products it is necessary to make products that will turn out to the best advantage. This is an acceptable alternative way of cooking this delicious cake.

PREPARATION TIME: 20 minutes • COOKING TIME: 40 minutes
(7 minutes in microwave)
Ground cinnamon (to sprinkle on pan)
Finely granulated white sugar (to sprinkle on pan)
1 large cooking apple
2 tablespoons butter or salt-reduced
monounsaturated margarine
1$\frac{1}{3}$ cups finely granulated white sugar
$\frac{1}{2}$ teaspoon vanilla extract
2 eggs, lightly beaten
$\frac{2}{3}$ cup low-fat milk
1$\frac{1}{3}$ cups gluten-free baking mix
$\frac{2}{3}$ cup white rice flour
$\frac{2}{3}$ cup brown rice flour
2 teaspoons gluten-free baking powder

1. Preheat oven to 350°F.

2. Prepare an 8-inch fluted cake pan by spraying with cooking spray. (If cake is to be cooked in the microwave, use a ring-shaped microwave-safe cake container.)

3. Sprinkle prepared pan with cinnamon and sugar.

4. Peel and thinly slice apple. Arrange apple slices in prepared pan.

5. Cream butter, sugar, and vanilla.

6. Gradually add egg to creamed mixture, beating well after each addition.

7. Stir in half the milk.

8. Sift baking mix, rice flours, and baking powder and stir into mixture and mix well.

9. Stir in remainder of the milk. Mixture should be a moist consistency.

10. Carefully spread mixture into prepared pan.

11. Place into a moderate oven and bake for approximately 35–40 minutes or until cooked in the center when tested.

OR Microwave on high for 5 minutes. Continue to microwave on medium for 2 minutes or until cooked when tested.

12. Leave in pan for 10 minutes before turning out onto a fine wire rack to cool.

BUTTER CAKE

My daughter made up this recipe for a plain butter cake. The best flavor is obtained by using butter; however, margarine can be used if desired.

PREPARATION TIME: 15 minutes • COOKING TIME: 40 minutes

$\frac{1}{2}$ cup butter or salt-reduced
monounsaturated margarine

1 cup sugar

$\frac{1}{2}$ teaspoon vanilla extract

2 eggs

2 cups gluten-free, plain, all-purpose flour

1$\frac{1}{2}$ teaspoons gluten-free baking powder

1 cup low-fat milk

1. Preheat oven to 325°F.

2. Prepare a 9-inch round, fluted ring cake pan by spraying with cooking spray.

3. Cream butter, sugar, and vanilla.

4. Add eggs one at a time, beating well after each addition.

5. Add sifted flour and baking powder. Mix well.

6. Stir in milk and spread into prepared pan.

7. Place into a moderate oven and cook for approximately 40 minutes or until cooked when tested.

8. When cooked, remove from oven and allow to cool in pan for 10 minutes before turning out onto a fine wire rack to cool.

CARROT CAKE

My great love for carrot cake led me to make up this recipe.
This delicious moist cake is best kept in the refrigerator.

PREPARATION TIME: 20 minutes • COOKING TIME: 50 minutes
(9 minutes in microwave)

$1\frac{1}{3}$ cups brown sugar

$\frac{1}{2}$ cup soft salt-reduced
monounsaturated margarine

4 cups grated carrot

$1\frac{1}{3}$ cups chopped walnuts

$1\frac{1}{3}$ cups chopped raisins

$1\frac{1}{3}$ cups gluten-free, plain,
all-purpose flour

$1\frac{1}{3}$ cups white rice flour

2 teaspoons cinnamon

2 teaspoons baking soda

$2\frac{2}{3}$ cups low-fat natural yogurt

1 teaspoon vanilla extract

1. Preheat oven to 350°F.

2. Prepare an 8-inch fluted ring cake pan by spraying with cooking spray.

3. Place all the ingredients into the large bowl of an electric food mixer. Mix on a low speed for 2 minutes or until the ingredients are well combined.

4. Pour mixture into prepared pan.

5. Place cake into oven and bake for approximately 50 minutes or until cooked when tested.

OR Microwave on high for approximately 9 minutes or until cooked when tested.

6. When cooked, remove cake from oven and leave in pan for 10 minutes, before turning out onto a fine wire rack to cool.

CHOCOLATE-ALMOND CAKE

I made this recipe for a special friend Aili for her name day. Aili is from Finland, and she tells me that it is more popular to celebrate name days in Finland, rather than birthdays. The flavor of this cake is improved if it is made the day before it is required. The cake is suitable to freeze.

PREPARATION TIME: 15 minutes • COOKING TIME: 1 hour

$\frac{1}{2}$ cup cocoa

$\frac{1}{2}$ cup hot water

$3\frac{1}{2}$ oz dark cooking chocolate, broken into small pieces

7 tablespoons unsalted butter, melted

$1\frac{3}{4}$ cups brown sugar

$\frac{2}{3}$ cup gluten-free self-raising flour

$\frac{2}{3}$ cup gluten-free, plain, all-purpose flour

5 oz ground almonds

$\frac{1}{2}$ teaspoon vanilla

4 eggs, separated

1. Preheat oven to 300°F.

2. Prepare an 8-inch round cake pan by spraying with cooking spray. Line pan with baking paper.

3. Combine cocoa and hot water in a large bowl. Stir until smooth.

4. Add chocolate, butter, brown sugar, flours, ground almonds, and vanilla. Stir until combined. It may be necessary to place into a moderately hot microwave for about 30 seconds to melt chocolate.

5. Beat in egg yolks, one at a time.

6. Place egg whites into a clean, dry bowl. Beat until stiff peaks form. Fold into chocolate mixture.

7. Pour into prepared pan.

8. Place into a moderate oven and bake for approximately 1 hour or until cooked when tested.

9. When cooked, remove from oven and leave in pan to cool.

10. Dust with gluten-free drinking chocolate or pure icing sugar before serving.

CHOCOLATE-BANANA CAKE

This is a very easy cake to make as it is mixed in a food processor. It is a delicious moist cake that is best stored in the refrigerator.

PREPARATION TIME: 15 minutes • COOKING TIME: 45 minutes

1 ripe banana

$\frac{1}{3}$ cup soy flour

$\frac{2}{3}$ cup brown rice flour

$\frac{1}{3}$ cup white rice flour

$\frac{1}{3}$ cup gluten-free corn flour

$\frac{1}{3}$ cup gluten-free custard powder

$\frac{1}{3}$ cup gluten-free, plain, all-purpose flour

$\frac{2}{3}$ cup cocoa

1 teaspoon baking soda

$1\frac{2}{3}$ cups brown sugar

1 cup canola oil

1 tablespoon white vinegar

$1\frac{1}{3}$ cups buttermilk

2 eggs

2 tablespoons strawberry jam

1 teaspoon vanilla extract

1. Preheat oven to 350°F.

2. Prepare a 9-inch round, fluted ring cake pan by spraying with cooking spray.

3. Peel banana and place into food processor.

4. Add remaining ingredients and blend until well combined.

5. Pour into prepared pan.

6. Place into a moderate oven and bake for 15 minutes. Reduce heat to 300°F for another 30 minutes or until cooked when tested.

7. Remove from oven and leave in pan for 10 minutes before turning out onto a fine-wire cake rack to cool.

CHOCOLATE MUD CAKE

This is a very dense, moist cake. It is best stored in the refrigerator.

PREPARATION TIME: 20 minutes • COOKING TIME: 75 minutes

1 cup butter or salt-reduced
monounsaturated margarine

5 oz dark cooking chocolate

$2\frac{2}{3}$ cups finely granulated white sugar

$1\frac{1}{3}$ cups hot water

1 tablespoon instant coffee

$\frac{1}{2}$ cup whiskey

$2\frac{1}{3}$ cups gluten-free, plain, all-purpose flour

3 tablespoons gluten-free self-raising flour

$\frac{1}{3}$ cup cocoa

2 eggs, lightly beaten

1. Preheat oven to 300°F.

2. Prepare a 9-inch square slab pan by lining with baking paper.

3. Combine butter, chocolate, sugar, water, and coffee in a microwave-safe bowl. Microwave on high for 1 minute and stir. Continue to microwave on high for 20-second intervals until chocolate is melted. Stir well.

OR Combine butter, chocolate, sugar, water, and coffee in a medium-sized saucepan. Stir over a gentle heat until chocolate is melted. Do not have the temperature too high or the chocolate will burn and be ruined. Stir well.

4. Allow mixture to cool.

5. Stir in whiskey.

6. Sift gluten-free plain and gluten-free self-raising flour and cocoa and stir into liquid.

7. Add lightly beaten egg and beat mixture well using an electric mixer.

8. Pour into prepared pan.

9. Place into a slow oven and bake for approximately $1\frac{1}{4}$ hours or until cake is cooked when tested.

10. Allow to remain in pan until cool.

DATE FUDGE SLICE

This slice has a delicious chocolate fudge texture. The dates may be omitted if desired or other dried fruit can be substituted for dates. The large soft dates that can be purchased loose at supermarkets or green grocers are used in this recipe.

PREPARATION TIME: 10 minutes • COOKING TIME: 30 minutes

$2/3$ cup finely chopped dates

7 tablespoons butter or monounsaturated
salt-reduced margarine

1 cup dark brown sugar

2 tablespoons cocoa

2 tablespoons treacle (such as Lyle's;
golden syrup can be substituted if desired)

1 egg, lightly beaten

$1/2$ teaspoon vanilla extract

$1\,2/3$ cups gluten-free self-raising flour

1. Preheat oven to 350°F.

2. Prepare a 7-inch square cake pan by spraying with cooking spray. Line base of pan with baking paper.

3. Combine dates, butter, sugar, cocoa, and treacle in a small saucepan. Cook over a low heat, stirring continuously until ingredients are well combined. Allow to cool.

OR Combine dates, butter, sugar, cocoa, and treacle in a small micro-wave-safe bowl. Microwave on high for 1 minute and stir. Microwave on high for another 1 minute and stir. Allow to cool.

4. Stir in egg, vanilla, and flour. Spread into base of prepared pan.

5. Place into a moderate oven and bake for approximately 30 minutes or until cooked when tested.

6. When cooked, remove from oven and allow to cool in pan. When cold, cut into small squares for serving.

GINGER CAKE

This is definitely a cake for those who like the flavor of ginger.

PREPARATION TIME: 15 minutes • COOKING TIME: 40 minutes

$\frac{1}{3}$ cup crushed gluten-free cornflake crumbs

7 tablespoons butter or salt-reduced
monounsaturated margarine

8 oz package light cream cheese

$1\frac{1}{3}$ cups finely granulated white sugar

$\frac{1}{2}$ teaspoon vanilla extract

3 eggs, lightly beaten

$2\frac{1}{3}$ cups gluten-free, plain,
all-purpose flour

1 teaspoon cinnamon

$\frac{1}{4}$ teaspoon ground cloves

$\frac{1}{4}$ teaspoon nutmeg

1 teaspoon ground ginger

$\frac{1}{3}$ cup finely chopped crystallized ginger

1 teaspoon baking soda

$\frac{1}{3}$ cup low-fat natural yogurt

1. Preheat oven to 350°F.

2. Prepare a 9-inch ring cake pan by spraying with cooking spray. Sprinkle gluten-free cornflake crumbs into pan.

3. Cream butter, cream cheese, sugar, and vanilla.

4. Gradually add eggs, beating well after each addition.

5. Sift flour and spices into creamed mixture and mix well. Stir in chopped ginger.

6. Stir baking soda into yogurt. Stir into cake mixture.

7. Spread into prepared pan.

8. Place into a moderate oven and bake for approximately 40 minutes or until cooked when tested.

9. When cooked, remove from oven and leave in pan for 10 minutes before turning out onto a fine wire rack to cool.

PECAN CAKE

Many people enjoy pecans in a cake.
If you do not have pecans, you can substitute walnuts.

PREPARATION TIME: 20 minutes • COOKING TIME: 35 minutes

2 tablespoons sunflower seed kernels

$\frac{1}{2}$ cup salt-reduced monounsaturated margarine

$\frac{2}{3}$ cup dark brown sugar

1 tablespoon honey

$\frac{1}{2}$ teaspoon vanilla extract

1 egg

$\frac{2}{3}$ cup chopped pecans

$1\frac{1}{3}$ cups chopped natural raisins

$\frac{2}{3}$ cup gluten-free, plain, all-purpose flour

$\frac{2}{3}$ cup white rice flour

1 teaspoon gluten-free baking powder

$\frac{1}{2}$ teaspoon baking soda

1 teaspoon cinnamon

$\frac{1}{3}$ cup rice bran

$\frac{2}{3}$ cup gluten-free instant infant rice cereal

1. Preheat oven to 350°F.
2. Prepare 8-inch fluted ring cake pan by spraying with cooking spray.
3. Sprinkle sunflower seed kernels into prepared pan.
4. Cream margarine, sugar, honey, and vanilla.
5. Add egg and mix well.
6. Stir pecans and raisins into creamed mixture.
7. Sift gluten-free flour, rice flour, baking powder, baking soda, and cinnamon into a small bowl. Stir in rice bran and rice cereal.
8. Stir dry ingredients into creamed mixture and mix well.
9. Spread mixture into prepared pan.
10. Place cake into oven and bake for approximately 35 minutes or until cooked when tested.
11. When cooked, remove from oven and leave in pan for 10 minutes before turning out onto a fine wire rack to cool.

PINEAPPLE CAKE

This is a moist cake. It is best stored in the refrigerator.
Serve hot or cold as desired with gluten-free custard or ice cream,
or use for Tropical Trifle (see page 142).

PREPARATION TIME: 10 minutes • COOKING TIME: 40 minutes
YIELD: 8 servings

6 tablespoons butter or salt-reduced
monounsaturated margarine

8 oz finely granulated white sugar

$\frac{1}{2}$ teaspoon vanilla extract

2 eggs

8 oz gluten-free self-raising flour

14 oz canned crushed pineapple
(drain and reserve juice)

8 tablespoons pineapple juice

1. Preheat oven to 350°F.

2. Prepare an 8-inch round cake pan by spraying with cooking spray. Line base of pan with baking paper.

3. Cream butter, sugar, and vanilla.

4. Lightly beat eggs. Gradually add to creamed mixture, beating well after each addition.

5. Sift flour and stir into mixture.

6. Stir in pineapple and pineapple juice.

7. Spread mixture into prepared pan.

8. Place into a moderate oven and bake for approximately 40 minutes or until cooked when tested.

9. Allow to cool in pan before turning out onto a fine wire rack.

Plain Cake (with Variations)

*My friend Alison has shared this recipe with me. It originated with
her friend Judy. The recipe is a memorial to Judy's son Michael,
who died in his early twenties. It now appears here, gluten-free.
At the bottom of the recipe are variations for added flavors.
It is an easy-to-mix cake that never seems to fail.*

PREPARATION TIME: 10 minutes • COOKING TIME: 30 minutes

1 cup sugar

2 eggs

1 1/3 cups gluten-free self-raising flour

1/2 cup soft butter or salt-reduced
monounsaturated margarine

1/3 cup milk

1 tablespoon gluten-free corn flour

1/2 teaspoon vanilla extract
or a few drops lemon extract

1. Preheat oven to 350°F.

2. Prepare an 8-inch round cake pan by spraying with cooking spray. Line base of pan with baking paper.

3. Wash bowl of an electric food mixer in hot water. (This is to allow the ingredients to mix together better.)

4. Place all the ingredients into the bowl. Beat on a slow-medium speed for 5 minutes. Pour into prepared pan.

5. Place into a moderate oven and bake for approximately 30 minutes or until cooked when tested.

6. Allow to stand in pan for 10 minutes before turning out onto a fine wire rack to cool.

Variations

Chocolate—Add 3 tablespoons cocoa and 5 oz melted chocolate.

Orange—Add finely grated rind of 1 orange and 1/3 cup orange juice in place of milk.

Nut—Add 1 cup finely chopped nuts of your choice.

Poppy Seed Cake

This is a delicious cake, liberally flavored with poppy seeds.

PREPARATION TIME: 20 minutes (+ 1 hour to soak poppy seeds)
COOKING TIME: 40 minutes

$\frac{1}{2}$ cup poppy seeds

1 cup low-fat milk

$\frac{1}{2}$ cup soft salt-reduced
monounsaturated margarine

1 teaspoon vanilla extract

$\frac{2}{3}$ cup finely granulated white sugar

2 eggs

1$\frac{1}{3}$ cups white rice flour

$\frac{2}{3}$ cup brown rice flour

$\frac{2}{3}$ cup gluten-free, plain,
all-purpose flour

$\frac{2}{3}$ cup gluten-free custard powder

2 teaspoons gluten-free baking powder

1. Soak poppy seeds in milk for 1 hour.

2. Preheat oven to 350°F.

3. Prepare a 9 x 5-inch loaf pan by spraying with cooking spray.

4. Place all the ingredients into the large bowl of an electric food mixer.

5. Mix on a low speed for 1 minute or until ingredients are well combined.

6. Pour mixture into prepared pan.

7. Place cake into oven and bake for approximately 40 minutes or until cooked when tested.

8. When cooked, remove from oven and leave in pan for 10 minutes before turning out onto a fine wire rack to cool.

SILVER CAKE

This cake is so named because only the whites of the eggs are used.

PREPARATION TIME: 15 minutes • COOKING TIME: 40 minutes

$\frac{2}{3}$ cup butter or salt-reduced
monounsaturated margarine

1 cup finely granulated white sugar

$\frac{1}{2}$ teaspoon vanilla extract

$\frac{2}{3}$ cup maize corn flour

$\frac{2}{3}$ cup low-fat milk

2 cups gluten-free, plain,
all-purpose flour

2 teaspoons gluten-free baking powder

2 egg whites

1. Preheat oven to 350°F.

2. Prepare an 8-inch fluted ring cake pan by spraying with cooking spray.

3. Cream butter, sugar, and vanilla.

4. Place corn flour into a small bowl. Add a little milk and blend well. Gradually stir in remaining milk.

5. Sift gluten-free plain flour and baking powder into a small bowl.

6. Gradually add corn flour liquid and sifted dry ingredients alternately to creamed mixture, mixing well after each addition.

7. In a separate, clean, dry bowl, beat egg whites until stiff and lightly fold into mixture.

8. Spread mixture into prepared pan.

9. Place cake into oven and bake for approximately 40 minutes or until cooked when tested.

10. When cooked, remove from oven and leave in pan for 10 minutes before turning out onto a fine wire rack to cool.

SPICY COFFEE CAKE

This cake is very easy to make and is high in fiber content.

PREPARATION TIME: 15 minutes • COOKING TIME: 45 minutes
(8 minutes in microwave)

1⅓ cups white rice flour

⅓ cup maize meal

⅔ cup gluten-free, plain, all-purpose flour

1 teaspoon gluten-free baking powder

½ teaspoon baking soda

¼ teaspoon cinnamon

½ teaspoon nutmeg

2 teaspoons instant coffee powder

6 oz brown sugar

1⅓ cups rice bran

⅔ cup polyunsaturated vegetable oil

1 cup cultured buttermilk

1 cup finely chopped raisins

1 egg, lightly beaten

1. Preheat oven to 350°F.

2. Prepare a 9-inch fluted ring cake pan by spraying with cooking spray.

3. Place all the ingredients into the large bowl of an electric food mixer.

4. Mix on a low speed for 1 minute or until all of the ingredients are well combined.

5. Pour mixture into prepared pan.

6. Place cake into oven and bake for approximately 45 minutes or until cooked when tested.

OR Microwave on high for approximately 8 minutes or until cooked when tested.

7. When cooked, remove from oven and leave in pan for 10 minutes before turning out onto a fine wire rack to cool.

ZUCCHINI CAKE

Dried fruits and pecans add to the delicious flavor of this cake.

PREPARATION TIME: 15 minutes • COOKING TIME: 45 minutes
(9 minutes in microwave)

$\frac{1}{2}$ cup salt-reduced monounsaturated margarine

$\frac{2}{3}$ cup raw sugar

$\frac{1}{2}$ teaspoon vanilla extract

2 eggs

$1\frac{1}{3}$ cups low-fat natural yogurt

$1\frac{1}{3}$ cups finely chopped natural golden raisins (sultanas)

$\frac{2}{3}$ cup finely chopped dried apricots

$1\frac{1}{3}$ cups grated zucchini

$\frac{2}{3}$ cup chopped pecans

$\frac{1}{3}$ cup sunflower seed kernels

$1\frac{1}{3}$ cups white rice flour

$1\frac{1}{3}$ cups gluten-free, plain, all-purpose flour

3 teaspoons gluten-free baking powder

1 teaspoon cinnamon

1. Preheat oven to 350°F.

2. Prepare a 9-inch fluted ring cake pan by spraying with cooking spray.

3. Cream margarine, sugar, and vanilla. Add eggs and mix well.

4. Stir yogurt, raisins, apricots, zucchini, pecans, and sunflower seed kernels into creamed mixture.

5. Sift rice flour, gluten-free flour, baking powder, and cinnamon into a small bowl.

6. Stir sifted dry ingredients into creamed mixture.

7. Spread mixture into prepared pan and smooth surface.

8. Place cake into oven and bake for approximately 45 minutes or until cooked when tested.

OR Microwave on high for approximately 9 minutes or until cooked when tested.

9. When cooked, remove from oven and leave in pan for 10 minutes before turning out onto a fine wire rack to cool.

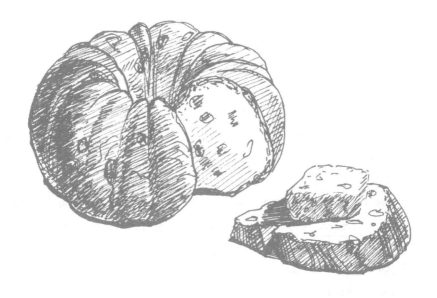

11.

Bread, Sweet Loaves, Muffins, and Extras

Bread

Multigrain Bread, 191

Potato-Rice Bread, 192

Almond Bread, 195

Brown and White Rice Bread, 196

Caraway Bread, 197

Cheese Bread, 198

Cheese and Tomato Bread, 199

Currant Bread, 200

Fruit Loaf, 201

Golden Bread, 202

Herb Bread, 203

Hi-Fiber Loaf, 204

Olive and Feta Bread, 205

Pine Nut Bread, 206

Plain Bread, 207

Rice Bread, 208

Spicy Raisin Bread, 209

Sweet Loaves

Apricot and Pineapple Loaf, 210

Jill's Date Loaf, 211

Marmalade-Date Loaf, 212

Pumpkin-Honey Loaf, 213

Muffins

Almond Muffins, 215

Apple and Apricot Muffins, 216

Apple Muffins, 217

Fruit Muffins, 218

Poppy Seed Muffins, 219

Pumpkin Muffins, 220

Spinach and Feta Muffins, 221

Sweet Potato and Tomato Muffins, 222

Extras

Carob Croissants, 223

Crumpets, 225

Easter Buns, 226

Focaccia, 228

Herb and Cheese Roll, 230

Peach Chutney, 231

Pikelets, 232

Pumpkin and Walnut Scones, 234

Scones, 236

BREAD

Making bread will be the most difficult task you will encounter as you explore the area of gluten-free cooking. The reason for this is that gluten is the elastic protein substance that stretches as a wheaten dough rises. When the product is baked, the gluten will set in its risen position. When there is no gluten in a bread product, it is difficult for it to rise. Do not be discouraged. It is possible to make gluten-free bread, but do not expect it to be the same as the wheaten product.

Making your own bread will allow you to have fresh bread that is free of artificial preservatives and is much cheaper.

Bread can be made using a wide variety of flour products other than wheaten flour. Rice flour, potato flour, soy flour, gluten-free flour, gluten-free bread mixes, and buckwheat flour are just a few of the possibilities.

Kitchen Scale

A kitchen scale is needed to make the bread recipes in this chapter. Using a scale allows for more precise measurement of dry ingredients, which is particularly important in bread making.

Bread Making (Baked in the Oven)

1. Deep-sided bread pans are best to use when making bread. The high sides on the pans encourage the bread to rise during the proving stage. Bread pans can be purchased at kitchen shops and are a worthwhile investment if you regularly make your own bread.

2. Grease bread pans thoroughly. You can sprinkle your greased pans with sesame or poppy seeds as desired.

3. Yeast is the raising agent used when making bread. It must be treated with care. Yeast requires the right conditions of warmth, moisture, food, and air to make it grow.

4. A bread dough must be proved (allowed to rise) in a warm place.

5. A commercially prepared bread mix contains a chemical raising agent which requires a temperature of 212°F to make it rise. The easiest way to do this is to turn your oven onto the lowest setting to allow the bread to rise. It is not necessary to remove the bread from the oven before increasing the temperature to bake the bread.

6. The addition of egg provides added protein and stability to the loaf.

7. The addition of a small amount of ascorbic acid (vitamin C) helps the dough to rise in the absence of gluten. One 25-milligram vitamin C tablet can be added to each recipe.

8. Crumbling can be a problem with some gluten-free breads. The addition of 1 or 2 tablespoons of polyunsaturated vegetable oil helps to bind the dough and makes the finished product less crumbly.

9. Remember that fiber is a very important part of your diet. Soy grits, polenta (also known as cornmeal), maize meal, brown rice flour, rice bran, and rolled rice flakes can be added to increase fiber. Rolled rice flakes can be made finer by crushing in a food processor or blender.

10. Fruit or sweet loaves can be made by adding your favorite natural dried fruit, for example raisins or dried apricots. Always finely chop dried fruit.

11. It is not a good idea to add too much spice to gluten-free bread as the addition of spice can make it more difficult for the bread to rise.

12. When making bread, it is necessary to mix the ingredients thoroughly. The ingredients must be thoroughly moistened with the liquid used.

13. A small amount of salt may be added if desired, although it is not essential.

14. It is an advantage when making bread to have the use of a heavy-duty mixer with a dough hook attachment. The dough can be mixed by hand of course—it just takes a little more effort.

15. Bread may be glazed to improve the appearance of the finished product. Use lightly beaten egg and a little milk and brush the bread before it is placed in the oven.

16. It is necessary to bake bread in a very hot oven. Reduce the heat after the first 10 minutes and continue to cook until the loaf is cooked when tested.

17. Buns can be an acceptable alternative to loaves. They seem to be more successful as they do not require as long a proving time and produce a more acceptable texture.

18. Gluten-free bread can be frozen for about 3 months.

19. It can be an advantage if you have an electric knife for slicing your homemade loaves.

20. Loaves will slice more easily if they are partly frozen. Freeze for approximately 1 hour before slicing, or allow a frozen loaf to thaw for approximately half an hour before slicing.

21. The best gluten-free bread results for the novice come by using a gluten-free commercial mix and adding your own gluten-free fiber. The addition of $2/3$ cup of the fiber mentioned in point 9 above to your favorite gluten-free commercial bread mix will produce a high-fiber loaf. Orgran makes excellent gluten-free bread mixes, as do other companies.

22. Croissants, buns, and scones are best freshened in the microwave oven for 10 seconds on high when required.

23. Last but by no means least, do not be discouraged by your first attempt. Gluten-free bread making is not easy. It takes time and practice to perfect the art!

MULTIGRAIN BREAD

*This bread is made from a number of different flours,
all of which are gluten-free. It has a very interesting flavor and
makes a delicious loaf of bread. The addition of polenta adds fiber.
The loaf has a close texture.*

1 tablespoon sesame seeds

4 tablespoons polyunsaturated margarine

2 tablespoons sugar

2 $\frac{1}{4}$-oz packets dried yeast

13 fl oz warm water

7 oz buckwheat flour

7 oz brown rice flour

7 oz gluten-free bread mix

7 oz polenta

1. Prepare a 2 lb (large) bread pan by greasing with some extra melted margarine. Sprinkle pan with sesame seeds.

2. Melt margarine and pour into a large bowl.

3. Stir in sugar, yeast, and water.

4. Allow to stand until mixture froths (approximately 10 minutes). Stir well.

5. Sift flours and bread mix into a medium-sized bowl. Add polenta and mix well.

6. Add dry ingredients to yeast liquid and mix well. Spread into prepared pan.

7. Heat oven to 212°F. Place bread into oven. Leave to prove for 20 minutes.

8. Leave bread in oven and increase oven temperature to 450°F. Bake for approximately 20 minutes. Reduce heat to 400°F and bake for another 10 minutes or until cooked when tested.

9. When cooked, remove from oven and leave in pan for 10 minutes before turning bread out onto a fine wire rack to cool.

POTATO-RICE BREAD

This bread has a close texture.
It is suitable for grilled snacks.

1 tablespoon sesame seeds
$\frac{1}{2}$ cup salt-reduced monounsaturated
margarine
2 $\frac{1}{4}$-oz packets dried yeast
2 cups lukewarm water
1 tablespoon sugar
8 oz potato flour
11 oz white rice flour

1. Prepare a 2 lb (large) bread pan by greasing with some extra melted margarine. Sprinkle pan with sesame seeds.

2. Melt margarine and place into a large mixing bowl.

3. Stir yeast into water. Add sugar and stir well. Pour liquid into bowl with margarine.

4. Allow to stand until mixture froths (approximately 10 minutes). Stir well.

5. Sift flours into a small bowl. Add flours to yeast liquid and mix well. Spread into prepared pan.

6. Heat oven to 212°F. Place bread into oven. Leave to prove for 20 minutes.

7. Leave bread in oven and increase oven temperature to 450°F. Bake for approximately 20 minutes. Reduce heat to 400°F and bake for another 10 minutes or until cooked when tested.

8. When cooked, remove from oven and leave in pan for 10 minutes before turning bread out onto a fine wire rack to cool.

Bread Making
(in an Electric Bread Maker)

Since the purchase of a bread maker, much fun and experimentation has occurred in my Country Kitchen to make delicious gluten-free bread.

When selecting a bread maker, there are a few points to keep in mind. It is important to choose a bread maker that is suitable for baking gluten-free bread. Select a brand with a shorter rather than longer cycle. The recipes in this section have been made using a machine that has a cycle of 2 hours and 20 minutes. As there is an absence of gluten in gluten-free bread, only a short cycle is necessary for gluten-free bread making. When selecting a bread maker with a short cycle, choose a brand to suit your needs. There can be some variations with different brand machines. Some experimentation may be necessary due to differences between appliances.

Here are some helpful points to keep in mind when making bread in an electric bread maker:

1. Water must be just warm, not too hot or it will kill the yeast.

2. Pour the liquid into the bowl of the bread maker first.

3. Thoroughly mix the dry ingredients together before adding to the liquid.

4. Dry ingredients can be warmed gently after mixing. Thoroughly mix again after warming.

5. Completely cover the liquid with the dry ingredients.

6. Sprinkle yeast over dry ingredients.

7. Set machine to the shortest setting according to the manufacturer's instructions.

8. At the end of the mixing cycle, just after the machine has shaped the bread, it is possible to remove the paddle. This will allow the loaf to cook without a hole where the paddle would have been if it had been left in the loaf while it was baking. This is a very useful idea when making gluten-free bread as it allows the loaf to be cut with greater ease.

9. Remove bread from machine at end of cycle. Leave in bowl.

10. Allow bread to sit in bowl for 10 minutes before turning out onto a fine wire rack to cool.

11. DO NOT at any stage be tempted to open the lid of the machine during the baking cycle. This could cause the bread to collapse.

12. Allow bread to cool completely before slicing. It is a good idea to partly freeze bread before slicing. This helps prevent it crumbling during slicing.

13. When packaging bread slices, separate with sheets of baking paper. This makes it easier to separate slices after it is refrigerated or frozen.

Some of the recipes in this section call for *xanthan gum*. Xanthan gum is available from supermarkets and health food stores. It is used to help the stability of the baked loaf. It is possible to make all the recipes without the addition of xanthan gum.

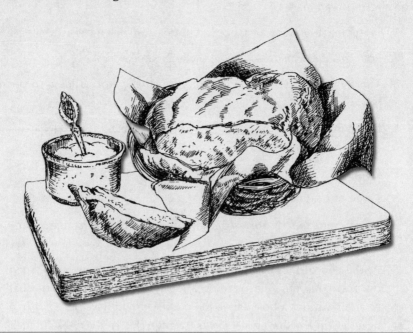

ALMOND BREAD

12 fl oz warm water

2 eggs

2 tablespoons canola oil

2 tablespoons golden syrup (such as Lyle's)

$\frac{1}{2}$ teaspoon vanilla extract

1 teaspoon white distilled vinegar

$3\frac{1}{2}$ oz white rice flour

8 oz brown rice flour

$1\frac{1}{2}$ oz potato flour

$1\frac{1}{2}$ oz polenta

5 oz gluten-free, plain, all-purpose flour

2 tablespoons brown sugar

3 tablespoons skim-milk powder

$1\frac{1}{2}$ oz sliced almonds

$1\frac{1}{2}$ oz diced almonds

$\frac{1}{4}$ teaspoon salt (optional)

1 teaspoon dried yeast

1. Pour warm water into a small bowl.

2. Add eggs and whisk well.

3. Stir in oil, golden syrup, vanilla, and vinegar. Pour into bread maker bowl.

4. Mix rice flours, potato flour, polenta, gluten-free flour, sugar, milk powder, sliced almonds, diced almonds, and salt (optional) well together.

5. Warm dry ingredients for 1 minute on high in the microwave oven. If you do not have a microwave oven, it is possible to put the dry ingredients into a bowl and stand the bowl over hot water, while stirring the dry ingredients.

6. Carefully put dry ingredients into bread maker bowl, taking care to completely cover the liquid.

7. Sprinkle yeast over dry ingredients.

8. Close lid and set machine to a short cycle according to directions with bread maker.

BROWN AND WHITE
RICE BREAD

This bread can be made dairy-free.

14 fl oz warm water

2 eggs

1 teaspoon white distilled vinegar

7 oz white rice flour

14 oz brown rice flour

3 tablespoons sugar

3 tablespoons skim-milk powder
(optional)

$\frac{1}{4}$ teaspoon salt (optional)

1 teaspoon dried yeast

1. Pour warm water into a small bowl.

2. Add eggs and whisk well. Stir in vinegar. Pour into bread maker bowl.

3. Mix rice flours, sugar, milk powder, and salt (optional) well together.

4. Warm dry ingredients for 1 minute on high in the microwave oven. If you do not have a microwave oven, it is possible to put the dry ingredients into a bowl and stand the bowl over hot water, while stirring the dry ingredients.

5. Carefully put dry ingredients into bread maker bowl, taking care to completely cover the liquid.

6. Sprinkle yeast over dry ingredients.

7. Close lid and set machine to a short cycle, according to directions with bread maker.

CARAWAY BREAD

14 fl oz warm water

2 eggs

1 teaspoon white distilled vinegar

$3\frac{1}{2}$ oz white rice flour

7 oz brown rice flour

10 oz gluten-free bread mix

3 tablespoons sugar

3 tablespoons skim-milk powder

1 tablespoon caraway seeds

$\frac{1}{4}$ teaspoon salt (optional)

1 teaspoon dried yeast

1. Pour warm water into a small bowl.

2. Add eggs and whisk well. Stir in vinegar. Pour into bread maker bowl.

3. Mix rice flours, gluten-free bread mix, sugar, milk powder, caraway seeds, and salt (optional) well together.

4. Warm dry ingredients for 1 minute on high in the microwave oven. If you do not have a microwave oven, it is possible to put the dry ingredients into a bowl and stand the bowl over hot water, while stirring the dry ingredients.

5. Carefully put dry ingredients into bread maker bowl, taking care to completely cover the liquid.

6. Sprinkle yeast over dry ingredients.

7. Close lid and set machine to a short cycle according to directions with bread maker.

CHEESE BREAD

14 fl oz warm water

2 tablespoons canola oil

1 large or 2 small eggs

$3\frac{1}{2}$ oz buckwheat flour

$3\frac{1}{2}$ oz polenta

7 oz brown rice flour

7 oz ground rice

2 tablespoons sugar

1 teaspoon gelatin

1 teaspoon xanthan gum (see page 194)

$\frac{1}{4}$ teaspoon salt (optional)

$\frac{2}{3}$ cup grated low-fat cheese

1 tablespoon parmesan cheese

1 teaspoon dried yeast

1. Pour warm water into a small bowl.

2. Pour in oil.

3. Add egg and whisk well. Pour into bread maker bowl.

4. Mix buckwheat flour, polenta, brown rice flour, ground rice, sugar, gelatin, xanthan gum, and salt (optional) well together.

5. Warm dry ingredients for 1 minute on high in the microwave oven. If you do not have a microwave oven, it is possible to put the dry ingredients into a bowl and stand the bowl over hot water, while stirring the dry ingredients.

6. Carefully put dry ingredients into bread maker bowl, taking care to completely cover the liquid.

7. Sprinkle cheeses and yeast over dry ingredients.

8. Close lid and set machine to a short cycle according to directions with bread maker.

CHEESE AND TOMATO BREAD

14 fl oz warm water

2 tablespoons canola oil

1 large or 2 small eggs

3½ oz Orgran gluten-free gourmet pesto
with tomato and linseed bread mix

3½ oz polenta

7 oz brown rice flour

7 oz ground rice

3½ oz finely chopped semi-dried tomatoes

2 tablespoons sugar

1 teaspoon gelatin

1 teaspoon xanthan gum (see page 194)

¼ teaspoon salt (optional)

⅔ cup grated cheese

1 tablespoon parmesan cheese

1 teaspoon dried yeast

1. Pour warm water into a small bowl.

2. Pour in oil.

3. Add egg and whisk well. Pour into bread maker bowl.

4. Mix gluten-free bread mix, polenta, brown rice flour, ground rice, tomatos, sugar, gelatin, xanthan gum, and salt (optional) well together.

5. Warm dry ingredients for 1 minute on high in the microwave oven. If you do not have a microwave oven, it is possible to put the dry ingredients into a bowl and stand the bowl over hot water, while stirring the dry ingredients.

6. Carefully put dry ingredients into bread maker bowl, taking care to completely cover the liquid.

7. Sprinkle cheeses and yeast over dry ingredients.

8. Close lid and set machine to a short cycle according to directions with bread maker.

CURRANT BREAD

14 fl oz warm water

2 tablespoons canola oil

1 large or 2 small eggs

4 oz buckwheat flour

4 oz polenta

7 oz brown rice flour

4 oz ground rice

$\frac{2}{3}$ cup currants

1 teaspoon cinnamon

$\frac{1}{4}$ teaspoon nutmeg

3 tablespoons sugar

1 teaspoon gelatin

1 teaspoon xanthan gum (see page 194)

$\frac{1}{4}$ teaspoon salt (optional)

1 teaspoon dried yeast

1. Pour warm water into a small bowl.

2. Pour in oil.

3. Add egg and whisk well. Pour into bread maker bowl.

4. Mix buckwheat flour, polenta, brown rice flour, ground rice, currants, cinnamon, nutmeg, sugar, gelatin, xanthan gum, and salt (optional) well together.

5. Warm dry ingredients for 1 minute on high in the microwave oven. If you do not have a microwave oven, it is possible to put the dry ingredients into a bowl and stand the bowl over hot water, while stirring the dry ingredients.

6. Carefully put dry ingredients into bread maker bowl, taking care to completely cover the liquid.

7. Sprinkle yeast over dry ingredients.

8. Close lid and set machine to a short cycle according to directions with bread maker.

FRUIT LOAF

14 fl oz warm water

2 tablespoons canola oil

1 large or 2 small eggs

4 oz buckwheat flour

4 oz polenta

7 oz gluten-free bread mix

4 oz ground rice

$\frac{1}{3}$ cup dried mixed fruit

1 tablespoon finely chopped dried apricot

1 tablespoon finely chopped dried apple

1 tablespoon finely chopped dried pineapple

1 tablespoon chopped peel

1 teaspoon cinnamon

$\frac{1}{4}$ teaspoon nutmeg

3 tablespoons sugar

1 teaspoon gelatin

1 teaspoon xanthan gum (see page 194)

$\frac{1}{4}$ teaspoon salt (optional)

1 teaspoon dried yeast

1. Pour warm water into a small bowl.

2. Pour in oil.

3. Add egg and whisk well. Pour into bread maker bowl.

4. Mix buckwheat flour, polenta, gluten-free bread mix, ground rice, mixed fruit, apricot, apple, pineapple, chopped peel, cinnamon, nutmeg, sugar, gelatin, xanthan gum, and salt (optional) well together.

5. Warm dry ingredients for 1 minute on high in the microwave oven. If you do not have a microwave oven, it is possible to put the dry ingredients into a bowl and stand the bowl over hot water, while stirring the dry ingredients.

6. Carefully put dry ingredients into bread maker bowl, taking care to completely cover the liquid.

7. Sprinkle yeast over dry ingredients.

8. Close lid and set machine to a short cycle according to directions with bread maker.

GOLDEN BREAD

11 fl oz warm water

2 eggs

2 tablespoons canola oil

2 tablespoons golden syrup (such as Lyle's)

1 teaspoon white distilled vinegar

7 oz brown rice flour

14 oz gluten-free bread mix

2 tablespoons brown sugar

3 tablespoons skim-milk powder

1 teaspoon xanthan gum (see page 194)

$\frac{1}{4}$ teaspoon salt (optional)

1 teaspoon dried yeast

1. Pour warm water into a small bowl.

2. Add eggs and whisk well.

3. Stir in oil, golden syrup, and vinegar. Pour into bread maker bowl.

4. Mix brown rice flour, gluten-free bread mix, sugar, milk powder, xanthan gum, and salt (optional) well together.

5. Warm dry ingredients for 1 minute on high in the microwave oven. If you do not have a microwave oven, it is possible to put the dry ingredients into a bowl and stand the bowl over hot water, while stirring the dry ingredients.

6. Carefully put dry ingredients into bread maker bowl, taking care to completely cover the liquid.

7. Sprinkle yeast over dry ingredients.

8. Close lid and set machine to a short cycle according to directions with bread maker.

HERB BREAD

14 fl oz warm water

2 tablespoons canola oil

1 large or 2 small eggs

$3\frac{1}{2}$ oz polenta

7 oz brown rice flour

7 oz ground rice

$3\frac{1}{2}$ oz Orgran gluten-free tomato
and linseed bread mix

1 teaspoon dried salad herbs

2 tablespoons sugar

1 teaspoon gelatin

1 teaspoon xanthan gum (see page 194)

$\frac{1}{4}$ teaspoon salt (optional)

1 teaspoon dried yeast

1. Pour warm water into a small bowl.

2. Pour in oil.

3. Add egg and whisk well. Pour into bread maker bowl.

4. Mix polenta, rice flour, ground rice, gluten-free bread mix, herbs, sugar, gelatin, xanthan gum, and salt (optional) well together.

5. Warm dry ingredients for 1 minute on high in the microwave oven. If you do not have a microwave oven, it is possible to put the dry ingredients into a bowl and stand the bowl over hot water, while stirring the dry ingredients.

6. Carefully put dry ingredients into bread maker bowl, taking care to completely cover the liquid.

7. Sprinkle yeast over dry ingredients.

8. Close lid and set machine to a short cycle according to directions with bread maker.

HI-FIBER LOAF

14 fl oz warm water

2 tablespoons canola oil

1 large or 2 small eggs

4 oz buckwheat flour

4 oz polenta

4 oz brown rice flour

$7\frac{1}{2}$ oz gluten-free bread mix

3 tablespoons sugar

1 teaspoon gelatin

1 teaspoon xanthan gum (see page 194)

$\frac{1}{4}$ teaspoon salt (optional)

1 teaspoon dried yeast

1. Pour warm water into a small bowl.

2. Pour in oil.

3. Add egg and whisk well. Pour into bread maker bowl.

4. Mix buckwheat flour, polenta, rice flour, gluten-free bread mix, sugar, gelatin, xanthan gum, and salt (optional) well together.

5. Warm dry ingredients for 1 minute on high in the microwave oven. If you do not have a microwave oven, it is possible to put the dry ingredients into a bowl and stand the bowl over hot water, while stirring the dry ingredients.

6. Carefully put dry ingredients into bread maker bowl, taking care to completely cover the liquid.

7. Sprinkle yeast over dry ingredients.

8. Close lid and set machine to a short cycle according to directions with bread maker.

OLIVE AND FETA BREAD

14 fl oz warm water

2 tablespoons canola oil

1 large or 2 small eggs

$3\frac{1}{2}$ oz Orgran gluten-free tomato and linseed bread mix

$3\frac{1}{2}$ oz polenta

7 oz brown rice flour

7 oz ground rice

$3\frac{1}{2}$ oz finely chopped olives of your choice

$3\frac{1}{2}$ oz finely chopped feta cheese

2 tablespoons sugar

1 teaspoon gelatin

1 teaspoon xanthan gum (see page 194)

$\frac{1}{4}$ teaspoon salt (optional)

$\frac{2}{3}$ cup grated cheese

1 tablespoon parmesan cheese

1 teaspoon dried yeast

1. Pour warm water into a small bowl.

2. Pour in oil.

3. Add egg and whisk well. Pour into bread maker bowl.

4. Mix gluten-free bread mix, polenta, brown rice flour, ground rice, olives, feta cheese, sugar, gelatin, xanthan gum, and salt (optional) well together.

5. Warm dry ingredients for 1 minute on high in the microwave oven. If you do not have a microwave oven, it is possible to put the dry ingredients into a bowl and stand the bowl over hot water, while stirring the dry ingredients.

6. Carefully put dry ingredients into bread maker bowl, taking care to completely cover the liquid.

7. Sprinkle cheeses and yeast over dry ingredients.

8. Close lid and set machine to a short cycle according to directions with bread maker.

PINE NUT BREAD

11 fl oz warm water

2 eggs

2 tablespoons canola oil

2 tablespoons golden syrup (such as Lyle's)

$\frac{1}{2}$ teaspoon vanilla extract

1 teaspoon white distilled vinegar

$10\frac{1}{2}$ oz white rice flour

$10\frac{1}{2}$ oz brown rice flour

2 tablespoons brown sugar

3 tablespoons skim-milk powder

1 teaspoon xanthan gum (see page 194)

1 teaspoon ground cinnamon

1 teaspoon mixed spice

$\frac{1}{2}$ teaspoon ground cloves

1 tablespoon poppy seeds

$3\frac{1}{2}$ oz golden raisins (sultanas)

$1\frac{1}{2}$ oz pine nuts

$\frac{1}{4}$ teaspoon salt (optional)

1 teaspoon dried yeast

1. Pour warm water into a small bowl.

2. Add eggs and whisk well.

3. Stir in oil, golden syrup, vanilla, and vinegar. Pour into bread maker bowl.

4. Mix rice flours, sugar, milk powder, xanthan gum, cinnamon, spice, ground cloves, poppy seeds, raisins, pine nuts, and salt (optional) well together.

5. Warm dry ingredients for 1 minute on high in the microwave oven. If you do not have a microwave oven, it is possible to put the dry ingredients into a bowl and stand the bowl over hot water, while stirring the dry ingredients.

6. Carefully put dry ingredients into bread maker bowl, taking care to completely cover the liquid.

7. Sprinkle yeast over dry ingredients.

8. Close lid and set machine to a short cycle according to directions with bread maker.

PLAIN BREAD

14 fl oz warm water

2 tablespoons canola oil

1 large or 2 small eggs

5 oz ground rice

4 oz polenta

5 oz brown rice flour

5 oz gluten-free bread mix

2 tablespoons sugar

1 teaspoon gelatin

1 teaspoon xanthan gum (see page 194)

$\frac{1}{4}$ teaspoon salt (optional)

1 teaspoon dried yeast

1. Pour warm water into a small bowl.

2. Pour in oil.

3. Add egg and whisk well. Pour into bread maker bowl.

4. Mix ground rice, polenta, brown rice flour, gluten-free bread mix, sugar, gelatin, xanthan gum, and salt (optional) well together.

5. Warm dry ingredients for 1 minute on high in the microwave oven. If you do not have a microwave oven, it is possible to put the dry ingredients into a bowl and stand the bowl over hot water, while stirring the dry ingredients.

6. Carefully put dry ingredients into bread maker bowl, taking care to completely cover the liquid.

7. Sprinkle yeast over dry ingredients.

8. Close lid and set machine to a short cycle according to directions with bread maker.

RICE BREAD

This recipe is designed for those who can have
no other grains except rice.

14 fl oz warm water

2 tablespoons canola oil

1 teaspoon white distilled vinegar
(optional)

10 oz white rice flour

10 oz brown rice flour

2 tablespoons sugar (optional)

2 tablespoons skim-milk powder
(optional)

$\frac{1}{4}$ teaspoon salt (optional)

1 teaspoon dried yeast

1. Pour warm water, oil, and vinegar into bread maker bowl.

2. Mix rice flours, sugar (optional), milk powder (optional), and salt (optional) well together.

3. Carefully put dry ingredients into bread maker bowl, taking care to completely cover the liquid.

4. Sprinkle yeast over dry ingredients.

5. Close lid and set machine to a short cycle according to directions with bread maker.

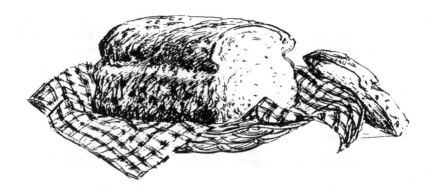

SPICY RAISIN BREAD

11 fl oz warm water

2 eggs

2 tablespoons canola oil

2 tablespoons golden syrup (such as Lyle's)

$\frac{1}{2}$ teaspoon vanilla extract

1 teaspoon white distilled vinegar

7 oz white rice flour

14 oz gluten-free bread mix

2 tablespoons brown sugar

3 tablespoons skim-milk powder

1 teaspoon xanthan gum (see page 194)

1 teaspoon ground cinnamon

1 cup natural golden raisins (sultanas)

$\frac{1}{4}$ teaspoon salt (optional)

1 teaspoon dried yeast

1. Pour warm water into a small bowl.

2. Add eggs and whisk well.

3. Stir in oil, golden syrup, vanilla, and vinegar. Pour into bread maker bowl.

4. Mix rice flour, gluten-free bread mix, sugar, milk powder, xanthan gum, cinnamon, raisins, and salt (optional) well together.

5. Warm dry ingredients for 1 minute on high in the microwave oven. If you do not have a microwave oven, it is possible to put the dry ingredients into a bowl and stand the bowl over hot water, while stirring the dry ingredients.

6. Carefully put dry ingredients into bread maker bowl, taking care to completely cover the liquid.

7. Sprinkle yeast over dry ingredients.

8. Close lid and set machine to a short cycle according to directions with bread maker.

SWEET LOAVES

These tasty sweet loaves are high in fiber and nutritious. They can be freshened for a few seconds in the microwave before required.

APRICOT AND PINEAPPLE LOAF

This is a very moist loaf with a delicious apricot and pineapple flavor. It is suitable for those on a low-fat diet.

PREPARATION TIME: **15 minutes** • COOKING TIME: **40 minutes**

$1\frac{1}{3}$ cups white rice flour

1 teaspoon gluten-free baking powder

1 teaspoon baking soda

4 tablespoons salt-reduced monounsaturated margarine

1 cup polenta

2 tablespoons finely granulated white sugar

$\frac{2}{3}$ cup chopped dried apricots

1 cup low-fat natural yogurt

$\frac{1}{2}$ teaspoon vanilla extract

$1\frac{1}{3}$ cups crushed pineapple (in natural juice)

1. Preheat oven to 350°F.

2. Prepare a 9- x 5-inch loaf pan by spraying with cooking spray. Line base with baking paper.

3. Sift rice flour, baking powder, and baking soda into a medium-sized mixing bowl.

4. Rub margarine into sifted dry ingredients until mixture resembles fine bread crumbs. This process may be done by hand or with the aid of an electric food processor.

5. Stir in polenta, sugar, and apricots.

6. Pour yogurt, vanilla, and pineapple into a small bowl and mix well. Stir liquid into dry ingredients.

7. Spread mixture into prepared pan.

8. Place loaf into oven and bake for approximately 40 minutes or until cooked when tested.

9. When cooked, remove from oven and leave in pan for 10 minutes before turning out onto a fine wire rack to cool.

JILL'S DATE LOAF

My friend Jill made me this lovely date loaf.
It slices very well and is suitable to freeze.

PREPARATION TIME: 10 minutes • COOKING TIME: 45 minutes

1$\frac{1}{3}$ cups chopped dates

$\frac{2}{3}$ cup golden raisins (sultanas)

$\frac{1}{2}$ cup chopped walnuts

4 tablespoons butter or salt-reduced monounsaturated margarine

1 cup brown sugar

1$\frac{1}{3}$ cups boiling water

1 egg, lightly beaten

$\frac{1}{2}$ teaspoon vanilla extract

2$\frac{2}{3}$ cups gluten-free self-raising flour

1 teaspoon bicarbonate soda

1 teaspoon cinnamon

$\frac{1}{2}$ teaspoon nutmeg

$\frac{1}{4}$ teaspoon ginger

1. Preheat oven to 350°F.

2. Prepare an 8$\frac{1}{2}$- x 4-inch loaf pan by spraying with cooking spray. Line base with baking paper.

3. Place dates, raisins, walnuts, butter, and sugar into a large mixing bowl. Add boiling water and mix until butter is melted. Allow to cool. Stir in egg and vanilla.

4. Sift flour, baking soda, and spices into fruit mixture and mix well.

5. Spoon mixture into prepared pan.

6. Place into a moderate oven and bake for 10 minutes. Reduce heat to 300°F. Bake for approximately 35 minutes or until cooked when tested.

7. When cooked, remove from oven and allow to cool in pan.

MARMALADE-DATE LOAF

*This loaf has the addition of marmalade
to give it a very nice flavor.*

PREPARATION TIME: **15 minutes** • COOKING TIME: **35 minutes**

1⅓ cups white rice flour

½ cup brown rice flour

⅓ cup maize corn flour

1 cup gluten-free, plain, all-purpose flour

2 teaspoons gluten-free baking powder

1 tablespoon brown sugar

1 tablespoon salt-reduced
monounsaturated margarine

1⅔ cups low-fat milk

2 tablespoons orange marmalade

1⅓ cups chopped dates

½ teaspoon vanilla extract

1. Preheat oven to 350°F.

2. Prepare an 8- x 4-inch loaf pan by spraying with cooking spray.

3. Sift flours and baking powder into a medium-sized mixing bowl. Stir in sugar.

4. Place margarine into a small saucepan and melt over a low heat.

OR Place margarine into a small microwave-safe bowl. Microwave on high for 20 seconds.

5. Stir milk, marmalade, dates, and vanilla into melted margarine.

6. Pour liquid into dry ingredients and mix well.

7. Spread mixture evenly into prepared pan.

8. Place loaf into oven and bake for approximately 35 minutes or until cooked when tested.

9. When cooked, remove from oven and leave in pan for 10 minutes before turning out onto a fine wire rack to cool.

PUMPKIN-HONEY LOAF

My friend Mary made me this lovely pumpkin-honey loaf.
It slices very well and is suitable to freeze.

PREPARATION TIME: **10 minutes** • COOKING TIME: **45 minutes**

5 oz gluten-free self-raising flour

5 oz white rice flour

2 teaspoons gluten-free baking powder

$\frac{1}{4}$ teaspoon baking soda

$\frac{1}{2}$ teaspoon mixed spice

$\frac{1}{4}$ teaspoon ground nutmeg

$\frac{1}{4}$ teaspoon ground cloves

$\frac{1}{4}$ teaspoon ground ginger

2 tablespoons skim-milk powder

2 tablespoons brown sugar

$\frac{2}{3}$ cup chopped dates

$\frac{2}{3}$ cup chopped walnuts

$\frac{1}{3}$ cup low-fat milk

$\frac{2}{3}$ cup creamed honey

4 tablespoons butter or salt-reduced
monounsaturated margarine

$1\frac{1}{3}$ cups cold, cooked, mashed pumpkin

2 eggs, lightly beaten

$\frac{1}{2}$ teaspoon vanilla extract

1. Preheat oven to 350°F.

2. Prepare an $8\frac{1}{2}$- x 4-inch loaf pan by spraying with cooking spray. Line base with baking paper.

3. Sift gluten-free self-raising flour, white rice flour, gluten-free baking powder, baking soda, mixed spice, ground nutmeg, ground cloves, ground ginger, and milk powder into a large bowl. Stir in brown sugar, dates, and walnuts.

4. Pour milk into a small microwave-safe bowl. Add honey. Microwave on high for 30 seconds and stir. Microwave for another 30 seconds. Add margarine and microwave for another 30 seconds. Stir in pumpkin, egg, and vanilla. Pour into dry ingredients in bowl and mix well.

5. Spoon mixture into prepared pan.

6. Place into a moderate oven and cook for 10 minutes. Reduce heat to 300°F. Bake for approximately 35 minutes or until cooked when tested.

7. When cooked, remove from oven and allow to cool in pan.

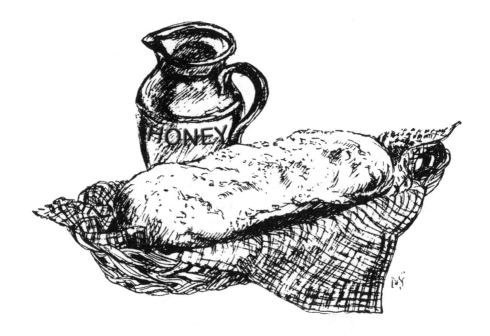

MUFFINS

Muffins are an excellent choice for gluten-free cookery. They are easy to make and can be a healthy, high-fiber addition to the diet. Muffins are best freshened in the microwave oven for 10 seconds on high when required.

ALMOND MUFFINS

PREPARATION TIME: 15 minutes • COOKING TIME: 12 minutes
YIELD: Approximately 20 muffins

$3\frac{1}{2}$ oz ground almonds

$\frac{1}{2}$ cup coconut

$\frac{1}{2}$ cup sugar

$\frac{1}{2}$ cup Orgran gluten-free self-raising flour

$\frac{1}{2}$ cup soft butter or salt-reduced monounsaturated margarine

3 eggs

$\frac{1}{3}$ cup almond flakes

1. Preheat oven to 440°F.

2. Prepare two 12-cup muffin pans by spraying with cooking spray. Line base of cups with baking paper circles.

3. Place ground almonds, coconut, sugar, and gluten-free self-raising flour into a medium-sized mixing bowl. Mix well.

4. Melt margarine and pour into dry ingredients in bowl.

5. Whisk eggs and stir into mixture.

6. Place tablespoons of mixture into prepared muffin tray.

7. Top with almond flakes.

8. Place into a hot oven and bake for approximately 12 minutes or until golden brown and cooked when tested.

9. When cooked, remove from oven and leave in tray for 5 minutes before placing muffins onto a fine wire rack to cool.

APPLE AND APRICOT MUFFINS

The combination of apple and apricot makes this a very tasty muffin recipe.

PREPARATION TIME: 12 minutes • COOKING TIME: 12 minutes

YIELD: Approximately 12 muffins

$1\frac{1}{3}$ cups brown rice flour

$1\frac{1}{3}$ cups gluten-free, plain, all-purpose flour

2 teaspoons gluten-free baking powder

$\frac{1}{2}$ teaspoon baking soda

$\frac{1}{2}$ cup sugar

1 apple, peeled and grated

$\frac{1}{3}$ cup finely chopped dried apricots

4 tablespoons salt-reduced monounsaturated margarine

1 egg, lightly beaten

$\frac{2}{3}$ cup low-fat natural yogurt

$\frac{1}{2}$ teaspoon vanilla extract

1. Preheat oven to 440°F.

2. Prepare a 12-cup muffin tray by spraying with cooking spray. Line base of cups with baking paper circles.

3. Sift rice flour, gluten-free plain flour, baking powder, and baking soda into a medium-sized mixing bowl. Add sugar, apple, and dried apricots and mix well.

4. Place margarine into a small saucepan and melt over a low heat. Allow to cool.

OR Place margarine into a small microwave-safe bowl. Microwave on high for 1 minute. Allow to cool.

5. Add egg, yogurt, and vanilla to melted margarine and stir well.

6. Pour liquid into dry ingredients and mix well.

7. Place tablespoons of mixture into prepared muffin tray.

8. Place muffins into a hot oven and bake for approximately 12 minutes or until golden brown and cooked when tested.

9. When cooked, remove from oven and leave in tray for 5 minutes before placing muffins onto a fine wire rack to cool.

APPLE MUFFINS

These are a wholesome treat for those who watch their nutrition intake.

PREPARATION TIME: 12 minutes • COOKING TIME: 12 minutes
YIELD: Approximately 12 muffins

1/3 cup white rice flour
1/2 cup brown rice flour
2/3 cup gluten-free, plain, all-purpose flour
1 teaspoon gluten-free baking powder
1/2 teaspoon baking soda
1/3 cup rice bran
1/2 cup sugar
1 apple, peeled and grated
4 tablespoons salt-reduced
monounsaturated margarine
1 egg, lightly beaten
1 1/3 cups low-fat natural yogurt
1/2 teaspoon vanilla extract

1. Preheat oven to 440°F.

2. Prepare a 12-cup muffin tray by spraying with cooking spray. Line base of cups with baking paper circles.

3. Sift rice flour, gluten-free plain flour, baking powder, and baking soda into a medium-sized mixing bowl. Stir in rice bran, sugar, and grated apple and mix well.

4. Place margarine into a small saucepan and melt over a low heat. Allow to cool.

OR Place margarine into a small microwave-safe bowl. Microwave on high for 1 minute. Allow to cool.

5. Add egg, yogurt, and vanilla to melted margarine and mix well. Pour liquid into dry ingredients and mix well.

6. Place tablespoons of mixture into prepared muffin tray.

7. Place muffins into a hot oven and bake for approximately 12 minutes or until golden brown and cooked when tested.

8. When cooked, remove from oven and leave in tray for 5 minutes before placing muffins onto a fine wire rack to cool.

FRUIT MUFFINS

These muffins have a lovely fruity flavor.

PREPARATION TIME: 12 minutes • COOKING TIME: 12 minutes
YIELD: Approximately 12 muffins

1⅓ cups gluten-free, plain,
all-purpose flour

⅔ cup white rice flour

2 teaspoons gluten-free baking powder

½ teaspoon baking soda

⅔ cup brown sugar

⅔ cup chopped dates

1 teaspoon finely grated orange rind

1 banana, well mashed

1 tablespoon finely chopped raw ginger

1⅓ cups cultured buttermilk

½ teaspoon vanilla extract

1. Preheat oven to 440°F.

2. Prepare a 12-cup muffin tray by spraying with cooking spray. Line base of cups with baking paper circles.

3. Sift flours, baking powder, and baking soda into a medium-sized mixing bowl. Stir in sugar, dates, and orange rind and mix well.

4. Place banana and ginger into a small bowl. Stir in buttermilk and vanilla and mix well.

5. Stir banana liquid into dry ingredients and mix well.

6. Place tablespoons of mixture into prepared muffin tray.

7. Place muffins into a hot oven and bake for approximately 12 minutes or until golden brown and cooked when tested.

8. When cooked, remove from oven and leave in tray for 5 minutes before placing muffins onto a fine wire rack to cool.

POPPY SEED MUFFINS

PREPARATION TIME: 12 minutes • COOKING TIME: 12 minutes
YIELD: Approximately 12 muffins

$\frac{1}{2}$ cup salt-reduced monounsaturated margarine

$\frac{2}{3}$ cup brown sugar

$\frac{1}{2}$ teaspoon vanilla extract

1 egg

$\frac{2}{3}$ cup cold, cooked, mashed pumpkin

$1\frac{1}{3}$ cups buckwheat flour

$\frac{2}{3}$ cup gluten-free, plain, all-purpose flour

$\frac{2}{3}$ cup brown rice flour

2 teaspoons gluten-free baking powder

$\frac{1}{2}$ cup poppy seeds

$1\frac{1}{3}$ cups low-fat natural yogurt

1. Preheat oven to 440°F.

2. Prepare a 12-cup muffin tray by spraying with cooking spray. Line base of cups with baking paper circles.

3. Cream margarine, sugar, and vanilla.

4. Add egg and beat well.

5. Stir pumpkin into creamed mixture.

6. Sift flours and baking powder into a small bowl. Stir in poppy seeds.

7. Stir dry ingredients and yogurt alternately into creamed mixture, mixing well after each addition.

8. Place tablespoons of mixture into prepared muffin trays.

9. Place muffins into a hot oven and bake for approximately 12 minutes or until golden brown and cooked when tested.

10. When cooked, remove from oven and leave in trays for 5 minutes before placing muffins onto a fine wire rack to cool.

PUMPKIN MUFFINS

*These muffins are very nutritious. They are suited to a special diet
which requires the omission of gluten, egg, and milk.
They are delicious when served warm.*

PREPARATION TIME: 15 minutes • COOKING TIME: 15 minutes
YIELD: Approximately 12 muffins

$\frac{1}{2}$ cup salt-reduced monounsaturated margarine
(milk-free)
$\frac{2}{3}$ cup brown sugar
$\frac{1}{2}$ teaspoon vanilla extract
$\frac{2}{3}$ cup cold, cooked, mashed pumpkin
$\frac{2}{3}$ cup white rice flour
$\frac{2}{3}$ cup potato flour
$\frac{2}{3}$ cup arrowroot
2 teaspoons gluten-free baking powder
$\frac{2}{3}$ cup ground rice
$\frac{2}{3}$ cup fresh orange juice
(approximately 1 large orange)

1. Preheat oven to 440°F.

2. Prepare a 12-cup muffin tray by spraying with cooking spray. Line base of cups with baking paper circles.

3. Cream margarine, sugar, and vanilla.

4. Stir pumpkin into creamed mixture.

5. Sift flours, arrowroot, and baking powder into a small bowl. Stir in ground rice.

6. Stir dry ingredients and orange juice alternately into creamed mixture, mixing well after each addition.

7. Place tablespoons of mixture into prepared muffin tray.

8. Place muffins into a hot oven and bake for approximately 15 minutes or until golden brown and cooked when tested.

9. When cooked, remove from oven and leave in tray for 5 minutes before placing muffins onto a fine wire rack to cool.

SPINACH AND FETA MUFFINS

PREPARATION TIME: **15 minutes** • COOKING TIME: **12 minutes**
YIELD: **Approximately 20 muffins**

3$\frac{1}{3}$ cups Orgran gluten-free self-raising flour

8 oz cooked spinach, shredded

5 oz low-fat feta cheese (with herbs)

$\frac{2}{3}$ cup chopped dried tomato

2 tablespoons finely chopped fresh dill

2 tablespoons parmesan cheese

6 tablespoons butter or salt-reduced
monounsaturated margarine

1 egg, lightly beaten

1$\frac{3}{4}$ cups natural low-fat yogurt

1. Preheat oven to 400°F.

2. Prepare two 12-cup muffin pans by spraying with cooking spray. Line base of cups with baking paper circles.

3. Place gluten-free flour, spinach, feta cheese, tomato, dill, and parmesan cheese into a large mixing bowl. Mix well.

4. Melt margarine and place into a medium-sized mixing bowl.

5. Stir in egg and yogurt and mix well.

6. Pour liquid into dry ingredients and mix well.

7. Place tablespoons of mixture into prepared muffin trays.

8. Place into a hot oven and bake for approximately 12 minutes or until golden brown and cooked when tested.

9. When cooked, remove from oven and leave in trays for 5 minutes before placing muffins onto a fine wire rack to cool.

SWEET POTATO AND TOMATO MUFFINS

These muffins are moist and are best stored in the refrigerator.
They are best not kept in the freezer.

PREPARATION TIME: 15 minutes • COOKING TIME: 15 minutes
YIELD: Approximately 12 muffins

2 eggs

$\frac{1}{3}$ cup olive oil

1 tomato

$1\frac{1}{3}$ cups finely diced cooked
sweet potato

$1\frac{1}{3}$ cups grated fat-reduced
cheddar cheese

$1\frac{1}{3}$ cups buttermilk

$2\frac{2}{3}$ cups Orgran gluten-free
self-raising flour

1 teaspoon gluten-free curry paste

Cracked black pepper, as desired

1. Preheat oven to 400°F.

2. Prepare a 12-cup muffin pan by spraying with cooking spray. Line base of muffin cups with baking paper circles.

3. Break eggs into a medium-sized mixing bowl. Add oil and whisk well.

4. Place tomato into boiling water. Leave for 2 minutes. Remove skin from tomato and finely dice.

5. Add tomato, sweet potato, cheese, buttermilk, gluten-free flour, curry paste, and pepper to mixing bowl and mix well. Mixture will be a moist consistency.

6. Place 2 heaping tablespoons of mixture into each prepared muffin-tray cup.

7. Place into a hot oven and bake for approximately 15 minutes or until golden brown and cooked when tested.

8. When cooked, remove from oven and leave in trays for 5 minutes before placing muffins onto a fine wire rack to cool.

EXTRAS

CAROB CROISSANTS

Croissants are delicious served warm for breakfast or as a snack.
Gluten-free yeast recipes require careful handling during preparation.

PREPARATION TIME: 50 minutes • COOKING TIME: 13 minutes
YIELD: Approximately 16 croissants

Croissants

$3\frac{1}{2}$ oz brown rice flour

$3\frac{1}{2}$ oz buckwheat flour

$3\frac{1}{2}$ oz rice flour

7 oz gluten-free bread mix

$\frac{1}{2}$ cup salt-reduced monounsaturated margarine

7 fl oz low-fat milk

$\frac{1}{4}$ oz packet dried yeast

2 tablespoons honey

2 tablespoons sugar

25 mg vitamin C tablet, crushed

Carob Spread

2 oz carob buttons (no added sugar)

1 oz maize corn flour

4 tablespoons water

2 tablespoons salt-reduced monounsaturated margarine

$\frac{1}{2}$ teaspoon vanilla extract

Croissants

1. Prepare a flat oven tray by spraying with cooking spray.

2. Sift flours and bread mix into a medium-sized mixing bowl and mix well.

3. Rub margarine into dry ingredients until mixture resembles fine bread crumbs. This process may be done by hand or with the aid of an electric food processor.

4. Place milk into a small saucepan. Heat over a low heat. Milk must be just warm, not hot.

OR Place milk into a small microwave-safe bowl. Microwave on high for approximately 40 seconds. Milk must be just warm, not hot.

5. Stir yeast, honey, sugar, and vitamin C into milk. Allow to stand until yeast froths in liquid (approximately 5 minutes).

6. Stir liquid into dry ingredients and mix well.

7. Turn dough out onto a lightly floured (gluten-free) board and knead lightly.

8. Divide mixture in half.

9. Roll each half into a flat circle, approximately 13 inches in diameter.

10. Cut each circle into 8 triangles.

11. Prepare carob spread.

Carob Spread

1. Place carob into a small double saucepan. Heat over a low heat until carob is melted.

OR Place carob into a small microwave-safe bowl. Microwave on medium-high for 30 seconds and stir. Continue to microwave on medium-high, stirring at 30 second intervals, until carob is melted.

2. Place corn flour into a small bowl. Add water and blend well. Stir into carob.

3. Stir in margarine and vanilla.

4. Stir over a low heat until carob mixture thickens.

OR Microwave on medium-high for 30 seconds and stir. Continue to microwave on medium-high, stirring at 30 second intervals, until carob mixture thickens.

To Combine

1. Preheat oven to 212°F.

2. Place a teaspoon of carob mixture in the center of the wide end of each triangle.

3. Carefully roll each triangle into a croissant shape.

4. Carefully place croissants onto prepared tray.

5. Place croissants into oven and leave to prove for 20 minutes.

6. Leave croissants in oven and increase oven temperature to 450°F. Bake for 10 minutes. Reduce heat to 400°F and bake for another 3 minutes or until golden brown and cooked when tested.

7. When cooked, remove from oven and leave on tray for 5 minutes before placing croissants onto a fine wire rack to cool.

CRUMPETS

I was asked to develop a crumpet recipe for a young lady who required a gluten-free diet. She told me she was delighted with the following recipe.

PREPARATION TIME: 15 minutes • COOKING TIME: 20 minutes
YIELD: Approximately 20 crumpets

2 teaspoons psyllium seed

$\frac{2}{3}$ cup warm water

$2\frac{2}{3}$ cups gluten-free self-raising flour

2 teaspoons dry yeast

$\frac{1}{2}$ teaspoon baking soda

$1\frac{1}{3}$ cups warm water

2 oz sugar

1. Place psyllium seed into $\frac{2}{3}$ cup warm water. Allow to stand for 5 minutes.

2. Place all the ingredients into a medium-sized mixing bowl and beat until mixture is a smooth consistency. This process can be done using an electric food processor and blending until smooth.

3. Heat an electric skillet to 340°F.

4. Place 4 egg rings into skillet. Spray egg rings and pan with cooking spray.

5. Place two tablespoons of mixture into each egg ring in skillet.

6. Cook until set on the surface. Turn and cook on reverse side until golden brown.

7. When cooked, remove crumpets from egg ring and place onto a fine wire rack to cool. Cover to prevent drying out.

8. Crumpets are best served toasted on the day they are made.

EASTER BUNS

Easter buns are a favorite at Easter time. They can be easily made so long as the conditions are right.

PREPARATION TIME: 45 minutes (includes proving time)
COOKING TIME: 15 minutes
YIELD: Approximately 15 buns

$\frac{1}{2}$ cup butter or salt-reduced
monounsaturated margarine

1 pint milk

$2\frac{1}{2}$ oz compressed yeast, finely crumbled,
or $2\frac{1}{2}$ oz packets of dehydrated yeast

$\frac{1}{2}$ cup sugar

$\frac{2}{3}$ cup golden raisins (sultanas)

2 lbs gluten-free, plain, all-purpose flour

1 teaspoon salt, as desired

Paste

$\frac{1}{3}$ cup gluten-free, plain, all-purpose flour

A little cold water

Glaze

$\frac{1}{2}$ teaspoon gelatin

$\frac{1}{3}$ cup cold water

1 tablespoon sugar

A couple of drops of lemon extract
(if desired)

Buns

1. For individual buns prepare two flat oven trays by spraying with cooking spray. For a batch of buns prepare a deep 12-inch square cake pan by spraying with cooking spray. Line base of pan with baking paper.

2. Melt butter. Add milk and warm to blood heat (about 98.6°F or 37°C). Do not overheat liquid.

3. Place yeast and sugar into a basin and stir well. Gradually stir in warm liquid. Allow to froth for a few minutes.

4. Pour yeast mixture into the bowl of a strong food mixer.

5. Add raisins and mix well.

6. Add gluten-free flour and salt. Mix well.

7. Cover basin with plastic film. Allow to prove in a warm place until mixture is twice its original size.

8. Remove plastic film and return to food processor and beat well to thoroughly mix dough.

9. Remove dough from bowl onto a lightly floured (gluten-free) board. Lightly flour hands with gluten-free flour. Take egg-sized portions and shape into individual buns.

10. Place buns onto preparing baking trays or into cake pan.

11. Put into a warm place to prove until buns are soft and springy.

12. Prepare paste for crosses.

Paste

1. Preheat oven to 400°F.

2. Mix flour and water to a stiff, smooth paste, taking care not to add too much liquid.

3. Using a small piping nozzle, or paper tube, pipe a cross on the top of each bun.

4. Place into a hot oven and bake for approximately 12–15 minutes or until golden brown and cooked.

5. Cool slightly and glaze while still warm.

Glaze

1. Soak gelatin in cold water. Place into a small saucepan and bring to a boil.

2. Stir in sugar.

3. Remove from heat and stir in lemon extract if desired.

FOCACCIA

The best results for focaccia are achieved by making up the dough and proving it in an electric bread maker. I find Orgran gluten-free, plain, all-purpose flour works best for focaccia. Focaccia is delicious cut into small pieces and dipped in olive oil and/or balsamic vinegar.

PREPARATION TIME: 40 minutes • COOKING TIME: 20 minutes
YIELD: 6–8 servings

1 cup warm water

2 tablespoons olive oil

1 teaspoon salt, as desired

2 teaspoons sugar

4 cups Orgran gluten-free, plain,
all-purpose flour

2 teaspoons dry yeast

$\frac{1}{2}$ teaspoon dried oregano

$\frac{1}{4}$ teaspoon dried basil

$\frac{1}{4}$ teaspoon dried rosemary

1. Prepare a large round pizza tray by spraying with olive oil spray.

2. Pour water and olive oil into the bowl of an electric bread maker.

3. Add the remaining ingredients.

4. Mix dough on the dough setting.

5. Press dough into prepared tray.

6. Cover loosely with plastic wrap. Place tray in a warm place to allow dough to rise. Dough should be soft and springy to touch. The temperature needs to be warm but not HOT for the dough to rise.

7. Preheat oven to 400°F. Place into a moderately hot oven and bake for approximately 20 minutes or until crusty and golden brown and cooked when tested. Test to see if the dough is cooked by inserting a fine wooden skewer in the center. If it comes out clean, the focaccia is cooked.

8. When cooked, remove from oven and allow to cool for 5 minutes before serving.

Variations

Dressed Focaccia

Prepare as for plain focaccia to point 7. Then brush top of dough after it has risen with 1–2 tablespoons olive oil. Top with a choice of sundried tomatoes, finely chopped olive, feta cheese, grated cheddar cheese, parmesan cheese, semi-dried bell pepper, finely chopped onion, finely chopped ham or bacon, finely chopped capers, finely chopped anchovies or sardines. Place into a moderately hot oven (400°F) and bake for approximately 20 minutes or until crusty and golden brown and cooked when tested. Test to see if the dough is cooked by inserting a fine wooden skewer in the center. If it comes out clean, the focaccia is cooked. When cooked, remove from oven and allow to cool for 5 minutes before serving.

Filled Focaccia

Prepare as for plain focaccia to point 4. Then press half the dough into the tray. Brush dough with olive oil. Spread fillings of your choice over the dough. Roll remainder of the dough and place over the fillings. Cover loosely with plastic warp. Place tray in a warm place to allow dough to rise. Dough should be soft and springy to touch. The temperature needs to be warm but not HOT for the dough to rise. Place into a moderately hot oven (400°F) and bake for approximately 20 minutes or until crusty and golden brown and cooked when tested. Test to see if the dough is cooked by inserting a fine wooden skewer in the center. If it comes out clean, the focaccia is cooked. When cooked, remove from oven and allow to cool for 5 minutes before serving.

HERB AND CHEESE ROLL

This roll is suitable to use for a light meal or as a savory snack.

PREPARATION TIME: 20 minutes • COOKING TIME: 20 minutes
YIELD: 8 servings

1⅓ cups white rice flour
2 teaspoons gluten-free baking powder
1⅓ cups Orgran gluten-free gourmet pesto
with tomato and linseed bread mix
¼ teaspoon dried mixed herbs
¼ teaspoon dried oregano
2 tablespoons salt-reduced monounsaturated margarine
1 cup cultured buttermilk
⅔ cup grated low-fat tasty cheese
1 tablespoon freshly grated parmesan cheese

1. Preheat oven to 425°F.

2. Prepare a flat oven tray by spraying with cooking spray.

3. Sift rice flour and baking powder into a medium-sized mixing bowl. Stir in gluten-free bread mix, mixed herbs, and oregano.

4. Rub margarine into dry ingredients until mixture resembles fine bread crumbs. This process may be done by hand or with the aid of an electric food processor.

5. Pour buttermilk into dry ingredients and mix to a firm dough.

6. Turn dough out onto a lightly floured (gluten-free) board and knead lightly.

7. Carefully and lightly roll out to a rectangle approximately 12 x 10 inches.

8. Sprinkle with cheeses.

9. Carefully roll up into a long roll starting at long side of rectangle.

10. Carefully place roll onto prepared tray.

11. Place roll into oven and bake for approximately 20 minutes or until golden brown and cooked when tested.

12. When cooked, remove from oven and leave on tray for 10 minutes before carefully placing roll onto a fine wire rack to cool.

PEACH CHUTNEY

Peach chutney is a family favorite,
especially when served with ham at Christmas.

PREPARATION TIME: 20 minutes • COOKING TIME: 35 minutes
YIELD: 4 x 10 fl oz jars

2 lbs peaches

1 large white onion,
peeled and finely diced

$\frac{1}{2}$ teaspoon cinnamon

$\frac{1}{4}$ teaspoon ground cloves

1 teaspoon ginger

$\frac{1}{2}$ teaspoon mixed spice

$\frac{1}{2}$ cup brown sugar

$\frac{1}{3}$ cup white distilled vinegar

Juice of 1 lemon

$\frac{1}{2}$ cup olive oil

$\frac{1}{3}$ cup sherry

1. Plunge peaches into boiling water. Allow to stand for 1 minute. Remove skins and finely dice peaches.

2. Place peaches, onion, cinnamon, cloves, ginger, spice, sugar, vinegar, lemon juice, and oil into a large saucepan.

3. Cook over a gentle heat until mixture thickens.

4. Stir in sherry. Cook for 1 minute.

5. When cooked, bottle in warm sterilized jars and seal.

PIKELETS

This recipe for pikelets—small, thick pancakes—has been a family favorite in our home for many years. A friend asked me to make up a gluten-free pikelet recipe.

PREPARATION TIME: 10 minutes • COOKING TIME: 20 minutes
YIELD: Approximately 24–30 pikelets,
depending on the individual size

2 eggs

$2/3$ cup finely granulated white sugar

$2/3$ cup low-fat milk

2 tablespoons butter or salt-reduced
monounsaturated margarine

$1/4$ teaspoon baking soda

$1/2$ teaspoon vanilla extract

$1^2/3$ cups Orgran gluten-free
self-raising flour

1. Separate eggs.

2. Place egg whites into a large dry, clean mixing bowl. Beat whites until they hold stiff peaks.

3. Gradually add sugar to egg whites, beating well after each addition.

4. Place egg yolks into a small bowl and beat well.

5. Stir egg yolks into egg white mixture, taking care not to overbeat or air will be removed from the egg-white mixture.

6. Pour milk into a jug.

7. Place butter into a small saucepan and melt over a gentle heat.

OR Place butter into a small microwave-safe bowl. Cover and microwave on high for 40 seconds or until butter is melted.

8. Pour melted butter into milk in jug. Stir in baking soda and vanilla.

9. Sift gluten-free flour into a medium-sized mixing bowl.

10. Add gluten-free flour and liquid alternately to the egg mixture, mixing well after each addition.

11. Heat an electric skillet to 340°F.

12. Spray skillet with cooking spray.

13. Place tablespoons of mixture into skillet.

14. Cook until bubbles appear on the surface. Turn and cook on reverse side until golden brown.

15. Place plastic wrap over a fine wire rack. When cooked, remove pikelets from skillet and place onto rack. Cover with plastic wrap to prevent drying out.

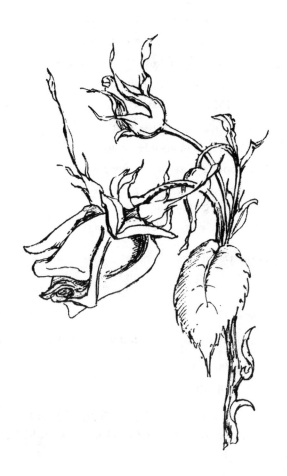

PUMPKIN AND WALNUT SCONES

It is possible to omit the walnuts
if plain pumpkin scones are required.

PREPARATION TIME: 20 minutes • COOKING TIME: 12 minutes
YIELD: Approximately 20 scones

4 tablespoons butter or salt-reduced
monounsaturated margarine

2 oz sugar

$\frac{1}{2}$ teaspoon vanilla extract

1 egg, lightly beaten

1$\frac{1}{3}$ cups cold, cooked, mashed pumpkin

$\frac{1}{2}$ cup finely chopped walnuts

$\frac{2}{3}$ cup milk

1$\frac{1}{3}$ cups white rice flour

1$\frac{1}{3}$ cups brown rice flour

$\frac{2}{3}$ cup potato flour

1$\frac{1}{3}$ cups gluten-free bread mix

2 teaspoons gluten-free baking powder

1 teaspoon Orgran gluten-free
gluten substitute

A little extra milk (for glazing)

1. Preheat oven to 400°F.

2. Prepare a 11- x 7- x 1$\frac{3}{4}$-inch oven tray by spraying with cooking spray.

3. Cream butter, sugar, and vanilla.

4. Gradually add egg to creamed mixture, beating well after each addition.

5. Mix in pumpkin and walnuts.

6. Gradually add milk and stir well.

7. Sift rice flours, potato flour, bread mix, baking powder, and gluten substitute into mixture and mix well. Mixture should be of a firm consistency.

8. Turn out onto a lightly floured (gluten-free) board and knead lightly. Pat out to 1-inch thickness.

9. Dip a $1\frac{1}{4}$-inch cutter in gluten-free flour. Cut out rounds and place onto prepared tray.

10. Glaze with a little extra milk.

11. Place into a hot oven and bake for approximately 12 minutes or until golden brown and cooked.

12. When cooked, remove from oven and leave on tray for 2 minutes. Place onto a fine wire rack to cool.

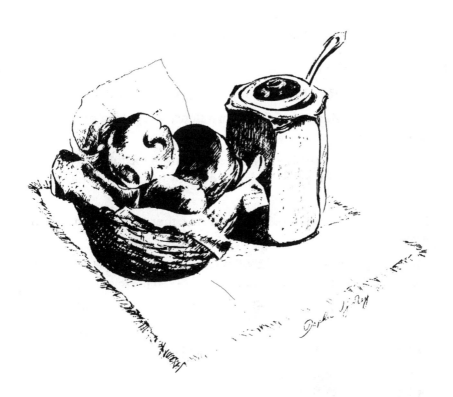

SCONES

When one cannot have gluten in the diet, a little
more thought is necessary to prepare a suitable scone recipe.

PREPARATION TIME: 15 minutes • COOKING TIME: 12 minutes
YIELD: Approximately 22 scones

$2\frac{2}{3}$ cups white rice flour

$2\frac{1}{3}$ cups Orgran gluten-free self-raising flour

$\frac{1}{3}$ cup maize corn flour

2 rounded teaspoons gluten-free baking powder

3 tablespoons salt-reduced
monounsaturated margarine

$2\frac{2}{3}$ cups low-fat milk

A little extra milk for glazing

1. Preheat oven to 440°F.

2. Prepare a 11- x 7- x $1\frac{3}{4}$-inch oven tray by spraying with cooking spray.

3. Sift rice flour, gluten-free flour, corn flour, and baking powder into a medium-sized bowl.

4. Rub margarine into sifted dry ingredients until mixture resembles fine bread crumbs. This process may be done by hand or with the aid of an electric food processor.

5. Pour milk into dry ingredients and mix thoroughly to form a firm dough.

6. Turn dough out onto a lightly floured (gluten-free) board and knead lightly. Pat out to $\frac{3}{4}$-inch thickness.

7. Cut out with a 2-inch floured (gluten-free) cutter and place onto prepared tray.

8. Glaze top of scones with a little extra milk.

9. Place scones into a hot oven and bake for approximately 12 minutes or until golden brown on top.

10. When cooked, remove from oven and leave on tray for 2 minutes before placing scones onto a fine wire rack to cool.

Glossary

ADDITIVES. There are a number of additives approved for use in the United States. These include thickeners, flavorings, and colorings. When the source is wheat or other grains that contain gluten, they are not gluten-free.

ANTI-CAKING AGENTS AND FREE-FLOWING AGENTS. These are used to ensure that powdered products flow freely. When the source is wheat or other grains that contain gluten, they are not gluten-free.

B VITAMINS. Whole-grain cereals are a major source of B vitamins. When cereals containing gluten are excluded from the diet, it is important to include other cereals high in the B vitamins. Soybeans and brown rice can be added to gluten-free diets to increase B-vitamin intake.

BAKING POWDER. Read labels carefully as some baking powders may contain ingredients that are not gluten-free. It is possible to make up your own gluten-free baking powder, with the following recipe:

Ingredients	$1\frac{1}{4}$ oz maize corn flour	$1\frac{1}{2}$ oz baking soda
	1 oz cream of tartar	1 oz tartaric acid
Method	1. Mix all the ingredients together.	
	2. Sift twice through a very fine sieve.	
	3. Store in an airtight container.	

BALANCED DIET. A balanced diet is one that provides all the nutrients (proteins, fats, carbohydrates, vitamins and minerals, and water) in the recommended quantities for good health.

BEER. Gluten-free beer is available in the United States. Check with your local supermarket or celiac society for further information.

BREAD. High-fiber (gluten-free) breads have good nutritional value. Gluten-free bread, sweet loaves, muffins, and scones can be freshened in the microwave for a few seconds just prior to serving. It can be easier to slice gluten-free bread if the loaf is partly frozen before slicing. Bread can be stored in the freezer for three months.

CALCIUM. Calcium is a mineral element generally best provided in the diet by dairy products. Calcium can also be obtained from canned salmon (plus bones), oysters, dark green vegetables, fresh fish, fortified-calcium soy drinks (check for gluten-free), and soybeans. Almonds and cashews also provide calcium in the diet, but considerable quantities are needed to provide the necessary daily calcium intake. Celiacs have a particular need to maintain their calcium intake throughout life. Poor calcium absorption prior to diagnosis increases the risk of osteoporosis (thinning bones) in celiacs, especially women.

CAUTION. It is necessary to exercise caution to avoid any traces of gluten when following a gluten-free diet. Sometimes people are still suffering symptoms when they think they have removed all traces of gluten from their diet. If symptoms do persist you should check with your doctor or dietitian as there may be a secondary intolerance (for example, soy).

CELIAC AWARENESS WEEK. October is celiac awareness week in the United States. The Celiac Sprue Association (CSA), its chapters, and resource units promote the overall awareness and meaning of celiac disease. Promotional literature can be obtained from CSA (www.csaceliacs.org).

CHOLESTEROL. Cholesterol is a waxy substance that the body produces. Excess cholesterol builds up in the arteries leading to the heart. This can commence from a very early age if a person follows incorrect eating habits.

COMMERCIAL GLUTEN-FREE FOODS. Information about gluten-free foods changes frequently. New product development and new technological advancements are occurring. The golden rule to remember is "When in doubt—leave out!" Do not consume a commercial product unless you are absolutely certain that the ingredients are gluten-free. Once you are diagnosed a celiac, it is important to become a member of a celiac society. You can then refer to the lists produced by the society, or seek advice from a dietitian.

COMPLEX CARBOHYDRATES. We should include more fruit, grains (gluten-free), breads (gluten-free), cereals (gluten-free), and vegetables in our diet to obtain complex carbohydrates. A gluten-free diet can be deficient in complex carbohydrates due to the removal of regular breads and cereals.

COOKIE CRUMBS. Collect crumbs from containers of gluten-free cookie and gluten-free cornflakes, and store in an airtight container. When a cookie crust is called for, a ready supply of gluten-free cookie crumbs is available.

CRISPBREADS. A variety of crispbread is available. One brand is Orgran. Their crispbreads are currently wheat and gluten-free, egg-free, dairy-free, yeast-free, and casein-free; however, always check labels carefully before purchasing. See www.orgran.com.

DAIRY PRODUCTS. These include milk, cheese, and yogurt. Read labels carefully to ensure the product is gluten-free.

DERMATITIS HERPETIFORMIS. This is a chronic skin disease requiring a gluten-free diet.

DIETARY FIBER. Dietary fiber, originally described as roughage in the diet, is the term used to describe a group of substances that are derived from plant cells (fruits, vegetables, grains, cereals, and nuts); includes pectins, lignins, gums, and other nondigestible carbohydrate matter.

Dietary fiber cannot be digested or absorbed in the human gastrointestinal tract but it stimulates the functioning of the colon. The fiber absorbs many times its weight in water and increases the volume of the stools passed, making for softer, easier elimination and the prevention of constipation. The inclusion of dietary fiber reduces the transit time of food through the gastrointestinal tract and so aids the body in eliminating waste products. Fiber plays a very important role in the way food affects body functions. It is credited with reducing the risk of some cancers, diverticulitis, hemorrhoids, and varicose veins. Fiber is very important when considering foods and planning healthy meals. It is an even more important consideration on a gluten-free diet, as valuable dietary fiber usually comes from wheat and oats.

Gluten-free diets can include polenta (also known as cornmeal), maize meal, soy grits, soybeans, and other beans such as kidney beans, cannellini beans, borlotti beans, garbanzo beans, mung beans, lentils, fresh fruits and vegetables, gluten-free muesli, gluten-free pasta, brown rice flour, rice bran, rolled rice flakes, ground rice, and psyllium seed to supply the much needed dietary fiber required by the body.

Ways of adding fiber to gluten-free diets include:

1. Use soy bran or rice bran. This can be added to cooking or sprinkled on breakfast cereals.

2. Use legumes such as beans, peas, and lentils in hamburgers, soups, casseroles, stews, and so on.

3. Serve gluten-free homemade muesli for breakfast. (See recipe page 32.)

4. Eat plenty of fruits and vegetables.

5. Use cracked buckwheat kernels in cooking.

6. Use rolled rice flakes.

DIETITIANS. A major dietary change of any kind should not be considered without a consultation with an accredited dietitian who has a good knowledge of celiac disease. A doctor or specialist can arrange a referral to a dietitian.

DINING OUT. Most chefs today have an understanding of special diets and will be pleased to assist with special dietary requirements (although it is a good idea to avoid restaurants that specialize in pasta and pancakes, unless you are sure they are gluten-free). If it is at all possible, phone ahead to discuss your gluten-free needs.

EGG SUBSTITUTES. These can be used to replace eggs in recipes. They have binding and raising properties that make them useful egg alternatives for special diets. Read labels carefully as some may contain gluten ingredients. The instructions for use can be found on the container.

Egg substitutes can be useful for:

1. Those who have to reduce their cholesterol levels

2. Those who are allergic to eggs

3. Those who do not wish to include animal products in their diet

4. Those on low-protein diets

5. Those on a diet restricted in phenylalanine (inability to metabolize phenylalanine is an inherited disease and causes phenylketonuria, PKU)

EXERCISE. This is necessary for a healthy lifestyle.

FLOURING BOARDS. Always use gluten-free flour for flouring boards.

GLUTEN. Gluten is the main protein in the cereal grains wheat, rye, barley, oats, and triticale. The amount of gluten in cereal grains varies markedly. Wheat (which ranges from 6 percent to 12 percent gluten) oats, barley, and rye are high in toxicity and must be avoided on a gluten-free diet. Sorghum and millet are gluten-free. Triticale is a hybrid developed by crossing wheat and rye and should be avoided on a gluten-free diet. Products made from wheat, rye, barley, oats, or triticale grain should be avoided.

GLUTEN-FREE GLUTEN SUBSTITUTE. A recently released Orgran product from Roma Foods. Gluten-Free Gluten Substitute mimics gluten and can be used in all gluten-free baking to increase workability.

GLUTEN-FREE SELF-RAISING FLOUR. You can make up your own gluten-free self-raising flour by adding 8 teaspoons baking powder (gluten-free) to 5⅓ cups of maize corn flour. Gluten-free flour mixes (for example, Orgran plain flour) can also be obtained from supermarkets and health food stores.

GLUTEN INTOLERANCE. Some people develop intolerance to gluten. This is different to celiac disease, but also requires a gluten-free diet.

GREASING COOKING DISHES. Cooking spray can be used for greasing cooking dishes, pans, or trays.

HAMBURGER PATTIES. When eating out, always check that hamburger patties are gluten-free. Meat patties can be contaminated by being cooked on a surface that has been used for cooking products coated with flour. Frying eggs for hamburgers can also transfer gluten in the same way.

ICING SUGAR. Pure icing sugar is finely ground sugar and is gluten-free. A product very similar to a commercially prepared pure icing sugar can be made at home with the aid of an electric blender or food processor. Place 8 ounces finely granulated white sugar into the bowl of a food processor and blend. The result will be a fine sugar powder, which can be used for cake icings in place of pure icing sugar.

Make your own gluten-free icing sugar. This can be made by mixing three parts of pure icing sugar with one part of maize corn flour. Store in an airtight container.

LABELING. The Food Allergen Labeling and Consumer Protection Act (FAL-CPA), which took effect January 1, 2006, requires foods containing milk, eggs, tree nuts, peanuts, shellfish, fish, soy, and wheat, to declare the allergen clearly on the ingredient list or by: (1) the word "contains" followed by the name of the major food allergen (milk, wheat, or eggs, for example); or (2) a parenthetical statement in the list of ingredients, for example "albumin (egg)." Further, the law requires the U.S. Food and Drug Administration (FDA) to finalize rules for the use of the term "gluten-free" on product labels by August 2008. (For more information, see the website of the American Celiac Disease Alliance: www.americanceliac.org.)

Always read the list of ingredients very carefully before purchasing products. If you want to confirm the suitability of ingredients you should check with an accredited dietition or celiac society in your area.

MAIZE MEAL. Maize kernels are ground coarsely to produce this meal. It is coarser than polenta (cornmeal). Maize meal is gluten-free.

MALT. Malt and malt products should not be included on a gluten-free diet. To produce malt, barley is steeped in water and allowed to germinate. The resultant product is not gluten-free. Malt can be produced from ingredients other than barley, for example rice; however, this is rare.

NUTRIENTS. Proteins, fats, carbohydrates, vitamins and minerals, and water make up the nutrients essential to life.

NUTRITION. Food and its relation to health.

NUTRITIONIST. An individual who studies the science of food and applies it to promote good health.

OBESITY. Obesity is defined as being more than 20 percent above the ideal weight recommended for a person's height. For children, age is also important.

ORGRAN. Orgran products are available at www.amazon.com and www.kitch-n-kaffe.com, as well as many natural food stores.

OVERWEIGHT. This is a state of carrying more weight than is recommended for your height, body build, and gender.

PASTA. Gluten-free pasta is widely available. See www.orgran.com for Orgran products. There are now a number of brands of gluten-free pastas on the market. A shorter cooking time is required for gluten-free pasta as there is no gluten present to hold the softened pasta together. Follow cooking instructions on the label.

POLENTA. Polenta is the Italian name for cornmeal. This is ground from the maize kernel. It is suitable for coarse breads. It can be used in recipes in place of cracked wheat. Polenta is excellent for adding fiber to the diet.

POTATO FLOUR. Potato flour can be used as a thickening agent, in cakes and sauces or gravies. It is most suitable to use in combination with soy flour.

PRODUCT AWARENESS. It is essential to become very astute when reading ingredient labels. Always check labels carefully before purchasing products.

RICE BRAN. It is very important to include fiber in a gluten-free diet. Rice bran meets this need, as well as providing excellent nutritional value for all diets. A nutritionally balanced, low-fat, high-fiber diet contributes to the prevention and control of diet-related diseases such as heart attack, diabetes, and bowel disorders, including constipation and colon cancer. Rice bran is a good source of protein, mono- and polyunsaturated fats, and dietary fiber. It contains the minerals magnesium, iron, and zinc, and the vitamins thiamine and niacin. It is totally free of cholesterol and gluten. Rice bran can absorb almost five times its bulk in liquid, making it an effective thickener for gravies, casseroles, sauces, and soups. It lends wholesome flavor and body to bread, cookies, cakes, muffins, and pies, and can also be sprinkled on breakfast cereals to add fiber and texture.

RICE FLOUR. Rice flour is gluten-free. It requires a little more liquid than equivalent quantities of wheat flour and has a slightly drier, more granular texture. It can be found in the flour section of supermarkets or health food stores.

SAUSAGES. Most sausages contain gluten products. Gluten-free sausages are available from most supermarkets and some butchers. Always check the ingredients carefully before purchasing. Remember that most sausages are high in fat and should be used sparingly in any diet.

SEAFOOD COMBINATIONS/SEAFOOD EXTENDER. Some seafood products such as crab sticks are held together with gluten ingredients. Some restaurants combine seafood ingredients such as crab sticks with fresh fish in dishes on the menu. Check carefully before ordering.

SEMOLINA. This is the granular starchy product obtained from the endosperm of hard wheat. Semolina flour is the fine floury part of the endosperm. It is not suitable for inclusion in a gluten-free diet.

SHORTENING FOR COOKING. Recipes in this book are made with polyunsaturated vegetable oil, mono/polyunsaturated margarine, peanut oil, olive oil, milk-free polyunsaturated margarine, and/or butter. Choices can be made to suit individual needs. Keep the quantity down to a minimum, wherever possible, as we are reminded to eat a diet low in fat.

SOY DRINK/SOY MILK. Calcium-fortified soy drink can be used in place of milk in recipes when a milk-free diet is chosen. Read labels carefully when planning a milk-free and gluten-free diet as some soy drinks contain gluten ingredients.

SOY FLOUR. Soy flour has a very strong, bitter taste when it is raw. This bitter flavor will be reduced with cooking, especially when combined with other gluten-free flours and sugar. Some celiacs have an intolerance to soy products.

STARCH. The term "starch" can be found on many manufactured products. It indicates a thickening or filling substance has been used in the product. Starch from sources such as potato, maize, or tapioca and those for which the source is unidentified are gluten-free. If the starch is from a gluten source, for example wheat, it should not be included on a gluten-free diet.

SWEETENERS. Nutritive sweeteners such as sugar, sucrose, sorbitol, and mannitol are gluten-free. They all contain energy and add calories to the diet. Nonnutritive sweeteners such as aspartame (Nutrasweet) are several hundred times sweeter than sugar. Care is necessary when they are found in manufactured products in a powdered form as they may contain gluten ingredients.

TAPIOCA. This is the starch prepared from the root of the cassava plant. The starch paste is heated to burst the granules. It is then dried in globules resembling sago. It is suitable to include in a gluten-free diet.

THICKENERS. Thickeners are added to foods to help improve the stability and texture, if required. Some thickeners and stabilizers are naturally derived from animal products, seaweed extracts, and vegetable gums. Others may be derived from wheat or other gluten-containing cereals and these should be avoided. Examples of gluten-free thickeners are: agar, alginates, corn, gelatin, guar gum, maize, pectin, potato, tapioca, unidentified thickeners, and xanthan gum.

TRAVELING. Gluten-free meals are available with some airlines. It is necessary to request a gluten-free meal when booking. It is a good idea to check the day before flying and when checking in to make sure gluten-free meals have been ordered. Indicate to the flight attendant when boarding the plane that a request for a gluten-free meal has been made. Care is necessary as some bread and condiments added to meals may not be gluten-free. If traveling overseas it is a good idea to travel with an up-to-date medical letter indicating special dietary requirements. This can save time at customs. It may be permissible to carry special gluten-free foods when entering and leaving some countries. It is a good idea to take a personal supply of gluten-free food when traveling overseas.

VEGETARIAN DIETS. People follow a vegetarian diet for various reasons. Whatever diet is followed, it is necessary to provide the body with the essential amino acids. These are the building blocks of proteins and cannot be manufactured by the body and must be supplied in the daily diet. This can be more difficult when following a vegetarian diet as the main source of essential amino acids is animal products. Amino acids are essential for growth and maintenance of good health.

Vitamin B_{12} must also be included in the diet. Animal products (for example, meats, eggs, dairy products) are the best source of vitamin B_{12}. Vegans (those who consume no animal products whatsoever) have to rely on foods that have been fermented to obtain vitamin B_{12}.

WATER. Water is an essential substance to life, second only to air in its importance. Aim for approximately eight glasses (4 pints) of fresh, clean water every day.

WHEAT FLOUR SUBSTITUTES. You can substitute one of the following in place of 1 cup of wheat flour:

1. $\frac{1}{2}$ cup maize corn flour plus $\frac{3}{4}$ cup soy flour

2. 1 cup soy flour plus $\frac{3}{4}$ cup potato starch

3. $\frac{3}{4}$ cup rice flour

4. 1 cup of Orgran (or other brand) gluten-free flour

WHISKEY. Whiskey is manufactured from the distillation of barley. The distillation process should ensure a gluten-free product. Rye whiskey and scotch whiskey have no detectable gluten.

WHERE TO BUY GLUTEN-FREE PRODUCTS. Leading retailers are now including a wider range of gluten-free products on their shelves. Most health food stores also carry a wide range of products. If the local supermarket does not carry the lines required, ask if they are happy to get products in for you.

XANTHAN GUM. This gum is used to give stability to gluten-free baked products. It is used with gluten-free flours, rice, maize, potato, tapioca, and soy. When gluten is taken out of a baked product it needs another substance to help give elasticity to the baked product. The amount of xanthan gum used in baked products varies. Generally speaking $\frac{1}{2}$ a teaspoon is used for a medium-sized cake like a banana loaf. One teaspoon is used for a pastry for a pie, and 1 teaspoon is used for a loaf of bread. If gum is stored in a cool, hygienic place it has a very long shelf life.

YOGURT. Yogurt is an excellent source of calcium. Check ingredients to ensure that it is gluten-free.

Index

Alcohol, 16
Alfalfa seeds, 16
Almond meal, 16
Almond Bread, 195
Almond Halva, 123–124
Almond Loaf, 144–145
Almond Muffins, 215
Almonds, 174
Amaranth, 16
Anzac Cookies, 158–159
Apple and Apricot
    Muffins, 216
Apple and Date Slice,
    170
Apple Crunch, 122
Apple Muffins, 217
Apple Slice, 169
Apple Tea Cake, 171–172
Apples, 6, 70
Apricot and Pineapple
    Loaf, 210
Apricots, 6, 216
Arrowroot, 17
Australian Coeliac, 5
Avocado, 46
Avocado Salad, 94

Baby rice cereal, 17
Baked Avocado with
    Crab, 46–47
Baked beans, 6
Baked Blueberry
    Cheesecake, 125–126
Baked goods, 157–185
Baked Omelette Roll,
    48–49
Baking powder, 17

Bananas, 6, 175
Barley, 17
Battered foods, 17
Bean mix, 6
Beans, 17
Beef, 56
Bell Pepper Soup, 40–41
Berry sauce, 132
Besan, 17
Beverages, 17
Blueberries, 125
Bran, 17
Bread making, electric,
    193–194
Bread mixes, commercial,
    18
Breads, 6, 9, 17, 188–209
Breakfast, 10, 29–37
Breast feeding, 9
Broccoli, 6, 79
Brown and White Rice
    Bread, 196
Brownies, 160
Buckwheat, 18
Buckwheat Pancakes, 30
Buns, 226
Butter and margarine, 18
Butter Cake, 172
Buttermilk, 18
Butterscotch sauce, 138

Cabbage, 6
Cakes, 18, 150, 167–185
Calcium, 3, 5, 10
Cancer, bowel, 3
Caramel color, 18
Caraway Bread, 197

Carob Croissants,
    223–225
Carrot Cake, 173
Carrots, 7, 66
Cassava, 18
Casseroles, 74, 80, 89,
    104, 106
CDF. *See* Celiac Disease
    Foundation.
CELIAC (listserve), 15
Celiac disease, 3–7, 10,
    13–23
    symptoms, 13
    testing for, 14
Celiac Disease
    Foundation (CDF),
    15
Celiac societies, 15–16
Celiac Sprue Association
    (CSA), 16
Celiac.com, 15
Celery and Lentil Soup,
    41
Cereals, 4, 6, 17
Cheese, 18, 198, 199, 230
Cheese and Tomato
    Bread, 199
Cheese Bread, 198
Cheesecake, 125
Cherries, 81
Cherry Chutney, 146
Chicken, 18, 77–86
    barbecue, 17
Chicken and Broccoli, 79
Chicken and Pineapple,
    83
Chicken Casserole, 80

Chicken in Red and
  White Wine, 77–78
Chicken with Cherry
  Sauce, 81–82
Chickpeas, 18
Chinese Beef, 56–57
Chocolate, 18, 147
Chocolate Brownies, 160
Chocolate Mud Cake,
  176
Chocolate Sauce
  Pudding, 127–128
Chocolate-Almond Cake,
  174
Chocolate-Banana Cake,
  175
Christmas Pudding,
  148–149
Chutney, 18, 21, 146, 231
Cinnamon, 166
Citrus, 86
Coconut, 18
Coconut Lime Chicken,
  84–85
Coconut Rice with Peach-
  Mango Purée, 128
Coffee, 18
Coffee cake, 184
Coffee Cream Cookies,
  161–162
Conversion tables, 26–27
Cookies, 18, 158–166
Corn, 7, 19
Corn chips, 19
Corn flour, 19
Corned beef, 19
Cornflakes, 19
Crab, 46
Crackers, 18
Cranberry Citrus
  Chicken, 86
Cream, 19
Cream cheese, 136
Croissants, 223
Crumble, 137
Crumpets, 225

CSA. See Celiac Sprue
  Association.
Cucumber Dressing, 96
Currant Bread, 200
Curried Lentil Pie,
  102–103
Curried Vegetable Soup,
  42
Curry, 19, 71
Custard, 19, 129
Custard Cookies, 163
Custard Pie, 130

Dairy, 4, 9, 18, 19, 21
Date Fudge Slice, 177
Dates, 138, 211, 212
Desserts, 121–142
Diet, gluten-free, 1–7,
  9–11, 13–23
Dips, 51, 64
Dressings, 95
Dumplings, 133
Easter Buns, 226–227
Easy Quiche, 57
Edna's Kisses, 164–165
Eggs, 19

Fats, 9
FDA. See U.S. Food and
  Drug Administration.
Festival Cake, 150–151
Feta, 109, 206, 221
Fiber, 6, 10
  counter, 6
Figs, 103
Fish, 9, 19
Flapjacks, 31
Flours, 19, 168
Focaccia, 228–229
Folic acid, 6
Fondant, 19
Food, 4, 9, 16–23
Food groups, 4, 6–7
Fruit, 4, 6, 9, 19. See also
  individual fruits.
Fruit in Grape Juice, 131

Fruit Loaf, 201
Fruit Mince Pies,
  151–153
Fruit Muffins, 218
Fruit Platter with Berry
  Sauce, 132
Fruitcake, 154–155
Fudge, 177

Garlic, 118
Gelatin, 19
Ginger Cake, 178
Glucose syrup, 19
Gluten, 3–7, 9–11, 13–23
Gluten-Free Mall, 16
GlutenSmart, 16
Glycemic index, 9
Golden Bread, 202
Golden syrup, 19
Golden Syrup
  Dumplings, 133
Grapes, 131
Gravy thickeners, 19
Greek Style Lasagna,
  58–59
Green and Gold Salad,
  96
Guar gum, 20
Guidelines for a Gluten-
  Free Lifestyle, 15

Halva, 123
Ham, 20
Ham Pie, 60–61
Hawaiian Pizza, 62–63
Herb and Cheese Roll,
  230
Herb Bread, 203
Herbs, 20
Hi-Fiber Loaf, 204
High fiber, 6
Holiday fare, 143–156
Honey, 20, 213
Honey Cookies, 165
Hydrolyzed vegetable
  protein, 20

Ice cream, 20
Icing sugar, 20
Intestines, 13–14
Iron, 3, 5, 10

Jam, 20
Jill's Date Loaf, 211

Lasagna, 58
Leeks, 104, 105
Legumes, 9, 20
Lemon Meringue Pie,
    134–136
Lentils, 7, 20, 103
Licorice, 20
Limes, 84, 118
Loaves, 144, 201, 204,
    210–214
LSA, 20
Lunch, 10
Lupins, 20

Main courses, 11, 55–91
Malt, 20
Maltodextrin, 20
Mango, 128
Manton, Maria, 3–7
Maple syrup, 20
Marinades, 20
Marmalade Date Loaf,
    212
Marzipan, 20
Mayonnaise, 21, 101
Meal plans, gluten-free,
    10–11
Meat, 4, 9, 21, 56–76
    deli, 19
Measurements, 26–27
Meatball Soup, 43–44
Meatballs with Yogurt
    Dipping Sauce, 64
Melon with Cream
    Cheese, 136
Meringue, 134
Microwaves, 28
Milk, 21

Millet, 21
Mince, 151
Molds, 50
Monosodium glutamate,
    21
Moussaka, 65–66
Muesli, 7, 32
Muffins, 215–222
Multigrain Bread, 191
Mushrooms, 98
Mustard, 21, 67

Noodles, 9
Nutrients, 5–6
Nuts, 21, 206

Oats, 21
Oils, 21
Olives, 21
Olive and Feta Bread,
    203
Olive and Fig Tapenade,
    103
Omelettes, 48
Oranges, 7, 66
Osteoporosis, 5
Oven temperatures, 28

Pancakes, 30–31, 33–34,
    36, 119
Pancakes with Raspberry
    Spread, 33–34
Pasta, 9, 21
Pastes, 21
Pâté, 52
Peach Chutney, 231
Peaches, 128
Peanut butter, 7, 21
Peanuts, 7
Pecan Cake, 179
Pickles, 21
Pies, 60, 68, 75, 87, 102,
    107, 110, 114, 116,
    130, 134, 151
Pikelets, 232–233
Pine Nut Bread, 206

Pineapple, 83
Pineapple Cake, 180
Pizza, 62
Plain Bread, 207
Plain Cake, 181
Polenta, 7, 21
Popcorn, 21
Poppy Seed Cake, 182
Poppy Seed Muffins,
    219
Poppy seeds, 21
Pork Chops with Carrot
    and Orange Sauce,
    66
Porridge, 35
Potatoes, 7
Potato and Leek
    Casserole, 104
Potato and Leek Slice,
    105
Potato and Mushroom
    Salad, 98
Potato Casserole, 106
Potato chips, 21
Potato Pie, 107
Potato Salad, 97
Potato Soy Bake, 108
Potato wedges, 21
Potato-Rice Bread, 192
Poultry, 9
Prawn Aspic Moulds,
    50–51
Pregnancy, 6
Psyllium, 22
Pudding, 127, 138, 148
Pumpkin, 7
    seeds, 22
Pumpkin and Feta
    Quiche, 109–110
Pumpkin and Walnut
    Scones, 234–235
Pumpkin Muffins, 220
Pumpkin-Honey Loaf,
    213

Quiche, 57, 109

Quinoa, 22

Resources, 15–16
Rhubarb and Strawberry
    Crumble, 137
Rib Steak with Mustard
    Sauce, 67
Rice, 7, 9, 22, 112, 128,
    196
    bran, 22
    flour, 22
Rice and Raisin Porridge,
    35
Rice Bread, 208
Rice cakes, 7
Ricotta Pancakes, 36
Rolls, 48, 230
Rye, 22

Sago, 22
Salads, 93–101
Salami, 22
Salmon, 53
Salmon Paté, 52
Salmon Pie, 87–88
Sardine Dip, 51
Sauces, 22, 66, 67, 70, 73,
    81, 138
Sausages, 22
Scones, 234, 236
Seafood, 87–91
Semolina, 22
Sesame seeds, 22
Shepherd's Pie, 68–69
Shortbread, 156
Silver Cake, 183
Slices, 169, 170, 177
Smoked Salmon Sushi,
    53–54
Snacks, 11
Sorghum, 22
Soups, 22, 39–54
Sourdough, 22
Soy, 22, 108

Soy sauce, 22
Spelt (flour), 22
Spices, 20
Spicy Coffee Cake, 184
Spicy Rice Bread, 209
Spinach and Feta
    Muffins, 221
Spinach Pie, 110–111
Spinach Salad, 99
Spinach Vegetable Rice,
    112–113
Starch, 22
Starters, 39–54
Steak with Apple and
    Wine Sauce, 70
Sticky Date Pudding with
    Butterscotch Sauce,
    138–139
Stir-fry, 117
Stawberries, 137
Stock, 22
Sugar, 23
Sultanas, 7
Sunflower seeds, 23
Sushi, 23, 53
Sweet Curry, 71
Sweet loaves, 210–214
Sweet Potato and Tomato
    Muffins, 222
Sweet Potato Salad, 100

Tabouli, 23
Taco sauce, 73
Taco shells, 23
Tacos, 72
Tamari, 23
Tapenade, 103
Tapioca, 23
Tarts, 140
Tea, 23
Tea cake, 171
Thickeners, 23
Tofu Mayonnaise, 101
Tomatoes, 199, 222

Tomato Pie, 114
Tomato Soup, 45
Treacle Tart, 140–141
Triticale, 23
Trifle, 142
Tropical Trifle, 142
Tuna Casserole, 89–90
Tuna Mornay, 91

U.S. Food and Drug
    Administration, 15

Vanilla, 23
Veal Casserole, 74
Veal Pie, 75–76
Vegetable Pie, 116
Vegetable Stir-Fry, 117
Vegetable-Rice Patties, 37
Vegetables, 4, 6, 9, 23,
    102–119. See also
    individual vegetables.
Villi, 13
Vinegar, 23
Vitamin C, 5

Walnuts, 234
Walnut-Cinnamon
    Cookies, 166
Water, 9
Water chestnuts, 23
Weight gain, 9
Wheat, 23
Wine, 70, 77
Worcestershire sauce, 23

Yeast, 23
Yeast extract, 23
Yogurt, 23, 64

Zinc, 5, 10
Zucchini Cake, 185
Zucchini Pancakes, 119
Zucchini with Lime and
    Garlic, 118

About the Author

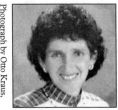

Photograph by Otto Kraus,
The Goulburn Studio

Ruby M. Brown is a qualified food technology educator who has worked with students in all areas of home economics. She is a talented and dedicated teacher and author. *Gluten-Free Cooking* is one of her books on special diets, the others being *Good Food for Diabetes* and *Milk-Free Cooking.* She has also written many textbooks and workbooks.